14.95

Research Team - Laboratoires Boiron

Jean Boiron - Jacky Abecassis - Philippe Belon

AF870224

ASPECTS OF RESEARCH IN HOMEOPATHY

Volume I - 1983

Editions Boiron

Translated by D. CLAUSEN - M.J. MAGNILLAT

All translation, reproduction and adaptation rights reserved for all countries including the U.S.S.R.
© Boiron, France, 1983 (Editions française)
© Boiron, France, 1984 (Translation)

ISBN 2.85742.011.0

FOREWORD

For over 30 years, we have contributed to research in the field of Homeopathy.

The great number of trials we carried out in University laboratories were communicated during national or international congresses.

Most of them were presented during the « Homeopathic Scientific Congress », an annual meeting of research people founded by Dr François Lamasson and myself in 1961.

Up to now, this research work has been published in the Annales Homéopathiques Françaises.

We felt it became indispensable to have the result of this research published more widely in order to meet the expectations of the medical and scientific world.

That is the goal of this new publication.

This first study deals only with pharmacological research.

However, clinical trials are presently being carried out and will be published in a forthcoming issue.

Jean Boiron
Doctor of Pharmacy, Bachelor of Science
General Secretary to the Research Committee
of the Liga Medicorum Homeopatica Internationalis.

This publication was conceived by the Research Team of Laboratoires Boiron who financed its undertaking, and defined the protocols in collaboration with the research workers.

We want to thank particularly :

Annie Bernard
Laboratory Assistant - the Central Laboratory of Biology - Hopital Debrousse - LYON

Jean-Claude Cazin
Professor of Pharmacodynamics - Law and Health College - LILLE University

Jean Cotte
Professor - Claude Bernard University - LYON 1 - Biologist, Hospital Department Head

Jean-Louis Gaborit
Research worker at the Pharmacodynamics Laboratory - Law and Health College - LILLE University

Jacques de Gerlache
Research worker - LOUVAIN Catholic University

Georges Halpern
Visiting Professor Children Hospital - STANFORD

Marc Lans
Research worker - LOUVAIN Catholic University

Henri Pacheco
Professor of Chemical Biology - National Institute of Applied Sciences - LYON

Marcel Roberfroid
Professor of Biochemistry - LOUVAIN Catholic University

Jean Sainte-Laudy
Head of PARIS Allergology and Immunology Laboratory.

TABLE OF CONTENTS

INTRODUCTION

From its very beginnings, Homeopathy claimed to be a medicine based on experience. Its indications and materia medica were all founded on experiments conducted with substances administered in infra-toxic doses to both healthy individuals (pathogenesies or provings) or sick ones (therapeutics).

Criticisms later directed against it were mainly centered around the idea that, at the level of potencies used, no active substances could no longer be traced in the administered remedies. Homeopaths therefore endeavored, by carrying out physico-chemical studies, to determine the height of potency up to which it was possible to substantiate the presence of a medically active substance, however weak its concentration may be.

More recently, homeopaths have themselves carried out, or have directed University teams to do so, a type of trial consisting of poisoning animals or plants of various species with different substances used in infra-lethal doses.

These trials presently constitute reliable examples of the activity of certain Hahnemanian potencies ; they have recently been extended to studies carried out in vitro with cell cultures, or in an a-cellular medium (resulting from cell-fractioning).

These experiments do not prove that the substances studied are medically active, but they do disprove the argument according to which they would be ineffective owing to the high potency level of the products.

Confident as they were that these facts would enable them to refute their detractors' chief argument, Homeopaths have initiated double blind clinical tests of their remedies. These tests, carried out according to a methodology in all respects comparable to the one used for the clinical study of other remedies, require the presence of a homeopathic physician, so as to make sure that the remedies are prescribed in accordance with the rules of Homeopathy.

The positive results of these trials have been published; other studies are presently being carried out both in France and abroad.

We cannot possibly attempt here to cover the whole range of research having been carried out in Homeopathy. We felt there was more interest in, first, situating the main lines of this research, and, second, to expone in detail certain specific projects with a particular attention to the evolution of methodologies. Research in Homeopathy has made use of several main types of methods, according to the conceptions and training of the searchers concerned.

Therapists: whether they be physicians or veterinarians, have collected a certain number of facts, observations and evidence regarding the effect of homeopathic remedies; this type of work, however, is not scientifically convincing, as it does not answer the problem of reproductibility or non-reproductibility of such reported facts.

Nevertheless, the accent must be put on work performed in the field of veterinary medicine: first of all because it refutes the argument of the placebo effect of the remedies, and second, because they were carried out upon a very large number of animals, thereby constituting a true series of trials in themselves.

Thus, a 10,000 bird hen farm was tested for the effect of a homeopathic complex designed to increase the birds' resistance to stress. Some industrial-type hen farms, for example, house tens of thousands animals cooped up in strictly artificial conditions. The birds are fed by food-conveyors, and eggs are collected automatically as they fall through a hole situated in the rear of the nest floor. Under such artificial conditions, the average number of eggs laid per layer amounts to 250 eggs a year. Laying reaches a peak by the end of several months and then gradually decreases: this decrease is supposed to be caused by stress.

When these birds were given the appropriate homeopathic cocktail, the average number of eggs laid went up to 257 a year. For the entire farm, this means an extra 70,000 eggs every year. This tendency to lay more is evidenced only towards the end of birds' life, thus corroborating the idea that it is, at least partially, due to a diminished stress upon the birds towards the end of laying time. The 70,000 eggs difference existing between the treated laying farms and the untreated ones is highly significant.

Besides the interest presented by this type of trial in the agricultural and food industry, it also greatly comes in favor of the non-placebo character of homeopathic remedies.

Homeopathic laboratories, for their own part, carried out a large number of pharmacological-type research work in the course of the past 30 years.

Simultaneously, manufacturing and control standard for the homeopathic remedies were defined by all manufacturers. This was an indispensable step towards giving trials reproductible basis.

This research work aimed at refuting criticism of Homeopathy, such criticism generally applying to the absence of quantifiable effects of the remedy, this being due to the infinitesimal quantities of active principles contained in the product. The main trials destined to refute this criticism were carried out with folliculin, copper sulfate, arsenic, alloxane, aconite, aconitine and mercury.

All these trials consisted in sub-poisoning the birds with the above-mentioned substance and treating these poisoned subjects with Hahnemanian potencies of these same substances. A detailed account of several of these trials is to be found further on.

Other research work was aimed at defining the homeopathic remedies way of action:

- *Some consisted in doing physical measurements: measurement of the dielectric constant, of the superficial tension, study of the Raman-Laser spectrum of Hahnemanian potencies, as compared to the corresponding solvents.*
- *Others were meant to evidence a pharmacological effect of the classical type: in these trials, the remedy was administered, either to the whole animal, or to a given organ, cell, or cellular fraction, and a precise parameter, supposed to vary according to the effect of the Homeopathic remedy, was then studied. Among these trials, let us quote trials carried out with IGNATIA, GELSEMIUM, PHYTOLACCA and HISTAMINUM.*
- *Other work consisted of specifically Homeopathic pharmacological demonstrations. In the latter cases, a Homeopathic treatment was administered to animals, organs and cells, the pathological attack of which had been brought about by a principle having no connection whatever with the Homeopathic remedy used.*

After this brief survey, and without the slightest pretention to being exhaustive, we now invite you to consider the following five trials.

Philippe Belon

In this work, the term "Hahnemanian potencies" is often used.

We feel we should give the following definition for it:

- Potencies are successive deconcentrations of basic substances of plant, animal or mineral origin, done either at the 1/10th or at 100th, followed by potentization carried out in accordance with the Hahnemanian technique.

SECTION I

ACTION OF HAHNEMANIAN POTENCIES UPON ARTIFICIALLY PRODUCED CANCER IN ANIMALS

INTRODUCTION

At the beginning of this report, we wish to make it quite clear that, in spite of its title, the following research work has not been intended with a therapeutic aim in view.

Its target was to establish an EXPERIMENTAL PHARMACOLOGICAL MODEL, designed to demonstrate the activity of HAHNEMANIAN POTENCIES.

This model was completed by Professeur Roberfroid, after several years of successive experimental protocols being used.

The selected procedure was to induce hepatocarcinoma in rats by use of a chemical carcinogen. The resulting pathological condition was studied both in check rats and in tested rats.

The main difficulty lay in the establishment of a protocol required for obtaining reproductible symptomatology without resorting to an overly high dose of the toxic agent (this would have made any type of therapeutic action impossible).

Trials conducted with experimentally created carcinogenesis showed that cancer could be induced chemically by a conjunction of two substances:

– A cancerogenic substance: we selected 2 AAF (Acetylaminofluorene).

– A "promoter": in other words, a non-cancerogenic substance, the presence of which, however, is capable of enhancing the cancerogenic action of the first substance: we selected Phenobarbital (PB).

MATERIAL AND METHOD

EXPERIMENTAL PROTOCOL

In order to obtain a statistically accurate analysis of the results, the trial had to be conducted with a number of animals totalling about one thousand.

At mid-July 1980, 1002 Sprague Dawley rats (aged 21-22 days), were given 2 AAF (Acetylaminofluorene) at the rate of 0.03% in their food over a period of 21 days. This amount of cancerogenic substance is quite sufficient for the given purpose, and will not cause any direct poisoning.

After 10 days of normal feeding, the animals were given the "promoter" (Phenobarbital) in their food in an amount of 0.5%. This was continued until the end of August 1981.

The animals were simultaneously divided into 4 batches, as follows:

- A first batch of 255 rats was given 9 C ARN;
- a second bath of 255 rats was given 9 C AAF;
- a third batch of 255 rats wad given 9 C Phenobarbital;
- a fourth batch of 237 rats was used as "control" batch, and was given 9 C potentized Water.

And finally, a group of 27 rats was used as a "check" batch and received no treatment whatsoever.

Classification of rats in the various batches

	9 C ARN	9 C 2 AAF	PB 9 C	Control 9 C H_2O
Tested Rats	161	170	175	156
Deaths	49	50	48	49
Rats still alive	31	27	29	23
Total/Initial number*	241/255	247/255	252/255	228/237

* *Note: the difference in number corresponds to rats having been sacrificed – and not tested – in order to find out at which stage tumors do appear.*

For all batches, the corresponding treatment was administered in a proportion of 14% of a Hahnemanian potency introduced in the animals' drinking water – this ad libitum – all throughout the experiment.

ANALYZED RESULTS

a) Mortality

Mortality is low, and equal in the various batches.

b) Weight of animals

The evolution of the animals' average weight shows no significant difference between groups.

c) Evolution of tumors

The main data resulting from the experiment are to be found in the following charts.

Charts I to IV show results obtained for each of the "control" batches: 9 C H_2O, 9 C PB, 9 C 2 AAF and 9 C ARN.

For each of the 11 slaughterings done between January 1981 and February 1982, the following data appear on the various charts:

- the number of rats sacrificed (Nb);
- the number of rats with Zymbal's tumors (tumors of the meatus acusticus) (ZT);
- the number of rats with no pathological signs (RAS);
- the number of rats with cystic damage (cysts);
- the percentage of animals showing signs of hepatic damage, this percentage being detailed so as to evidence both the number of animals with benign hepatic damage and the number of animals with malignant hepatic damage;
- the number of rats with tumors of a non-hepatic origin (N He).

The number of rats tested is not necessarily equal to the total number of intoxicated rats plus the number of unharmed rats, as there are possibilities of inter-destruction among the animals.

Chart I

2 C H_2 O Control batch								
Month	**Nb**	**ZT**	**RAS**	**Cysts**	**% hepat. damage**	**Benign**	**Malign**	**NHe**
January	13	2	10	1	15	2	–	–
February	11	4	10	–	0	–	–	1
April	18	4	7	1	55	10	–	–
May	10	2	4	2	40	4	–	–
June	15	3	7	2	40	5	1	–
August	10	0	3	1	30	2	1	3
September	8	2	2	1	37	1	2	2
November	18	7	3	5	50	1	8	1
December	30	0	5	1	76	13	10	1
January	8	2	3	0	37	1	2	2
February	15	3	0	0	80	3	9	3
Total	**156**	**29**	**54**	**14**		**42**	**33**	**13**
%		**18.5**	**34.6**	**8.9**		**26.9**	**21.1**	**8.3**

Chart II

9 C PB batch								
Month	Nb	ZT	RAS	Cysts	% hepat. damage	Benign	Malign	NHe
January	9	2	8	1	0	–	–	–
February	12	6	10	1	0	–	–	1
April	17	2	10	2	29	5	–	–
May	15	3	9	1	33	5	–	–
June	15	2	9	–	33	5	–	1
August	15	3	9	3	20	2	1	–
September	9	7	6	2	0	–	–	1
November	28	9	9	3	32	5	4	7
December	30	0	5	2	73	13	9	1
January	10	4	6	2	20	–	2	–
February	15	1	8	3	13.3	–	2	2
Total	**175**	**39**	**89**	**20**		**35**	**18**	**13**
%		**22.3**	**50.9**	**11.4**		**20**	**10.3**	**7.4**

Chart III

9 C 2 AAF batch								
Month	Nb	ZT	RAS	Cysts	% hepat. damage	Benign	Malign	NHe
January	12	2	12	–	0	–	–	–
February	10	2	8	–	20	2	–	–
April	16	1	5	2	56	9	–	–
May	15	2	8	3	26	4	–	–
June	19	6	7	3	42	6	2	1
August	15	5	6	1	46	5	3	1
September	5	3	1	1	40	2	–	1
November	23	6	6	4	26	3	3	7
December	30	1	7	2	63	12	7	2
January	10	3	2	1	50	1	4	2
February	15	1	3	1	66	4	6	1
Total	**170**	**32**	**65**	**18**		**47**	**25**	**15**
%		**18.8**	**38.2**	**10.6**		**27.6**	**14.7**	**8.8**

Chart IV

9 C ARN batch								
Month	**Nb**	**ZT**	**RAS**	**Cysts**	**% hepat. damage**	**Benign**	**Malign**	**NHe**
January	10	0	7	1	20	2	–	–
February	10	3	9	–	10	1	–	–
April	16	0	7	4	31	4	1	–
May	15	0	4	3	53	7	1	–
June	15	3	9	1	33	4	1	1
August	15	3	8	2	27	3	1	1
September	5	4	4	–	20	–	1	–
November	21	10	9	6	24	3	2	1
December	30	0	5	5	63	12	7	1
January	8	4	3	1	37	2	1	1
February	16	2	1	1	56	3	6	5
Total	**161**	**29**	**66**	**24**		**41**	**21**	**9**
%		**18**	**40.9**	**14.9**		**25.5**	**13**	**5.6**

Chart V gives a global statistical synthesis. For each of the various batches: H_2O, PB, 2 AAF and ARN batches, it indicates:

– the initial number of rats;

– the percentage of RATS STILL ALIVE in February 1982 (this number is insignificant however, since it stands for the number of rats left alive after the successive slaughterings);

– the percentage of rats having died of SPONTANEOUS DEATH (this percentage being lower in the case of the Phenobarbital batch);

– the number of TESTED RATS, with an indication of those having died of ZYMBAL'S TUMOR;

– the percentage of unharmed rats: 34.6% for the "control batch" (treated with 9 C Potentized Water), 50.9% for the PB batch (a highly significant difference, considering the equality probability is 0.003), 38.5% for the 2 AAF batch (this being insignificantly different from the "control batch" and 40.9% for the ARN batch (a significant percentage, the equality probability being 0.24);

– facing this, the number of CONTAMINATED RATS stands as complement to 100 of the percentage of unharmed rats.

Percentages of rats suffering from hepatic damage are as follows:

- 48% for the H_2O batch;
- 30.3% for the PB batch (a significant figure, the equality probability being: 0.0013);
- 42.3% for the 2 AAF batch (insignificant percentage);
- 38.5% for the ARN batch, with an equality probability of 0.08).

THESE HEPATIC DAMAGES ARE THEN DETAILED INTO:

- **Percentages of benign damage**

- 26.9% for the H_2O batch;
- 20% for the PB batch (equality probability: 0.0013);
- 27.6% for the 2 AAF batch (insignificant value);
- 25.5% for the ARN batch (insignificant value).

- **Percentages of malignant damage**

- 21.1% for the H_2O batch;
- 10.3% for the PB batch (this figure is highly significant as the equality probability is: 0.0065);
- 14.7% for the 2 AAF batch (equality probability: 0.12);
- 13% for the ARN batch (equality probability: 0.06).

Chart V

Statistical synthesis				
Results	**H_2O**	**PB**	**2 AAF**	**ARN**
Initial number of rats	228	252	247	241
% Rats still alive	10.1	11.5	10.9	12.8
% Death	21.5	19	20.2	20.3
Number of rats tested	156	175	170	161
% ZT	18.5	22.3	18.8	18
% Without hepatic damage	34.6	50.9	38.2	40.9
% With hepatic damage	65.4	49.1	61.5	59.1
% Cysts	8.9	11.4	10.6	14.9
% Non hepatic neoplasms	8.3	7.4	8.8	5.6
% Hepatic damage	48	30.3	42.3	38.5
of which: benign	26.9	20	27.6	25.5
: malignant	21.1	10.3	14.7	13

Note: order of priority is as follows: hepatic damage > non-hepatic neoplasm > cyst.

The following graph is a graphical representation of the percentage of contaminated rats with reference to the duration of the experiment for the different batches.

When analyzing this graph, it becomes obvious that:

- the PB batch is at all times significantly different from the "control batch";
- the 2 AAF potencies batch is not significantly different from the "control batch";
- the ARN potencies batch proves to be significantly different only half-way through the experiment.

Graphical representation

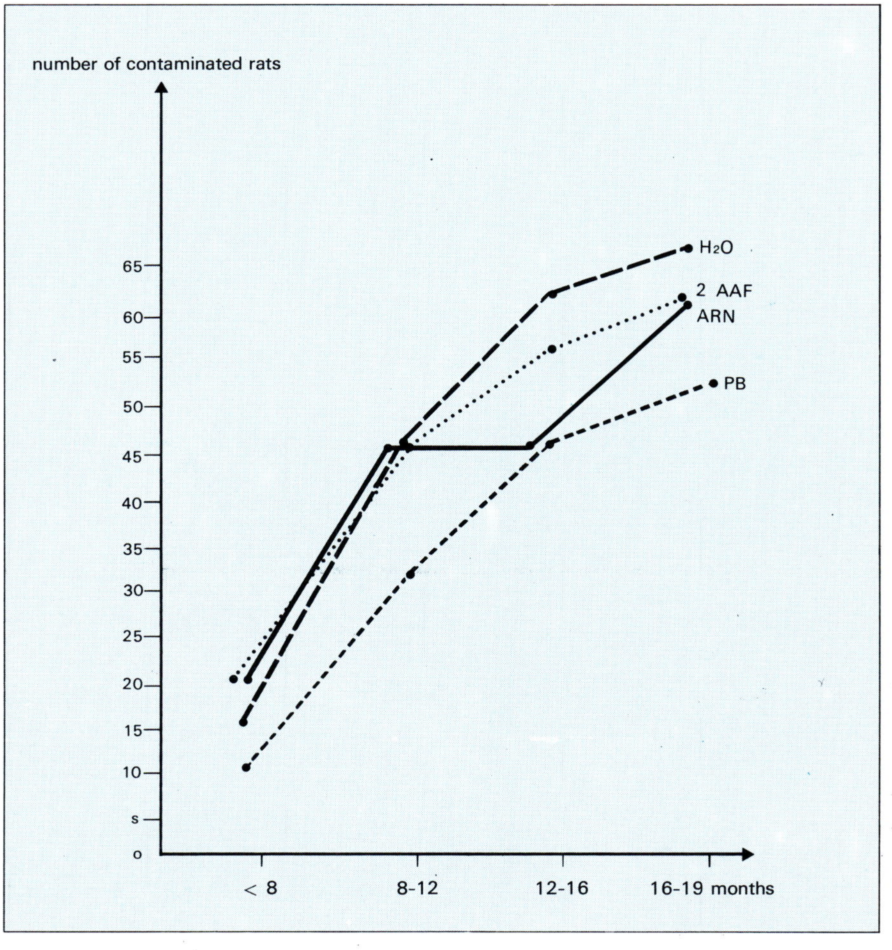

CONCLUSION

Several conclusions can be drawn from these trials. We, first of all, want to warn you against concluding that a homeopathic remedy can cure cancer.

As a matter of fact, experiments conducted have only succeeded in slowing down (in the case of RNA) and reducing (in the case of Phenobarbital) the appearance of chemically-induced carcinoma.

The only unquestionable scientific conclusion is that the administration of a 9 C Phenobarbital homeopathic treatment (at a theoretic rate of 400 molecules per ml of drinking water) PREVENTED THE APPEARANCE OF CHEMICALLY-INDUCED MALIGNANT CARCINOMA, IN HALF THE CASES.

This is a REMARKABLE DEMONSTRATION OF THE ACTIVITY OF A HAHNEMANIAN POTENCY, considering the large number of animals involved in this trial.

In Rats, the protective effect of 9 C PHENOBARBITAL on a Phenobarbital-induced hepatocarcinoma (0.5% in food) is positive. It is statistically significant by 0.0013%.

SECTION II

A PHARMACOLOGICAL STUDY OF THE RETENTION AND MOBILIZATION OF ARSENIC, AS CAUSED BY HAHNEMANIAN POTENCIES OF ARSENICUM ALBUM

INTRODUCTION

The elimination of a toxic element having previously been fixed in the system through the action of homeopathic potencies of this same element first observed in Guinea-Pig with arsenic and bismuth by Lapp and Wurmser, was confirmed in Pigeon with arsenic and antimony by Cier and Jean Boiron.

Mouriquand and Jean Boiron were also able to relate the elimination provoked by exogenous toxic products to the variations of vestibular chronaxy as considered as an objective control element of arsenical and antimoniated impregnation at a sub-toxic dose.

Cier and Jean Boiron had studied the specificity of this action in 1962, by researching whether there existed crossed reactions between arsenic and antimony, as these elements are chemically close to each other and have closely related biological properties.

As these tests had been highly positive, we decided to perform them again with a modernized protocol according to which arsenic is administered per os to all rats at time 0 (To).

Two experimental models have been selected:

- in the first test, the one and only injection of a Hahnemanian potency is given at To + 12 h, and the effect is measured 8 hours later;
- in the second test, injections of a Hahnemanian potency are given at To + 12 h, To + 24 h, To + 36 h, and rats are sacrificed at To + 7 days.

First test "in vivo":
effects of a single injection
of a Hahnemanian potency

MATERIAL AND METHOD

In this experiment, we tested the effects of a single injection of a Hahnemanian potency with 60 rats to which we administered a toxic solution of radio-active arsenic per os at time zero (To).

30 rats were TREATED with a 7 C Arsenicum Album potency, which was administered intra-peritoneally TWELVE HOURS AFTER INTUBATION, the other 30 rats having been TREATED with a 7 C Dynamized Water potency under the same conditions.

The rats had been distributed into metabolism cages immediately after injection; they were sacrificed EIGHT HOURS LATER when blood samples were taken from the hearts.

The 60 rats used were male Wistar strain rats with a weight of approximately 70 grams.

The toxic solution of radio-active arsenic was administered per os in a proportion of 0.5 ml/20 g of weight, in the following composition:

As_2O_3 (Prolabo arsenious anhydride): 10 mg/kg (roughy 700 µg per rat).

– ^{73}As (Amersham): 100 µCi/kg.

in a 5% gum syrup.

An injection of 1 ml of a Hahnemanian potency, from Laboratoires Boiron was given to each rat.

Metabolism cages are metallic cages equipped with glass devices separating the urine and the feces.

The counting device used for quantitative analyses, and the counting device used for gamma radiations bears the INTERTECHNICS trademark from Centre Oscar Lambret.

ANALYZED RESULTS

1. WITH BLOOD

A difference (Chart I) is to be observed between blood concentrations of arsenic in rats treated with 7 C Arsenicum Album and blood concentrations of arsenic in rats treated with 7 C Potentized Water.

This is evidenced 8 hours after the administration of the Hahnemanian potency: rats having received 7 C Arsenicum Album display an average blood concentration of 8.65 µg As/100 mg blood, while rats treated with 7 C Potentized Water display an average blood concentration of 9.15 µg As/100 mg blood.

Chart I

Blood concentrations measured at T_0 + 20 h. in rats treated with Hahnemanian potencies at T_0 + 12 h.
(results in µg of arsenic for 100 mg blood)

7 C Arsenicum Album

– 8.61	– 7.87	– 7.99	– 8.65	– 8.77	– 8.08
– 8.72	– 8.77	– 8.80	– 9.27	– 8.46	– 8.79
– 8.98	– 9.20	– 8.69	– 7.58	– 9.07	– 9.22
– 7.66	– 9.02	– 9.33	– 9.60	– 6.77	– 9.52
– 8.17	– 9.02	– 8.05	– 9.48	– 8.80	

General average = 8.65 ± 0.66

7 C Potentized Water

– 8.12	– 8.24	– 8.49	– 10.84	– 9.79	– 10.48
– 9.28	– 10.11	– 9.33	– 8.42	– 9.54	– 9.44
– 8.94	– 7.62	– 8.99	– 9.56	– 9.09	– 9.25
– 8.93	– 9.51	– 9.02	– 9.47	– 9.08	– 8.95
– 8.96	– 9.52	– 8.55	– 8.64		

General average = 9.15 ± 0.69

(Fisher-Snedecor and Student's Test)

THIS DIFFERENCE, with a higher figure for rats treated with 7 C Arsenicum Album, existing between blood concentrations in arsenic of both 30 rats populations treated under the same conditions with different Hahnemanian potencies IS SIGNIFICANT WITH AN ACCURACY RATE OF 99% ($P. < 0.01$).

On the diagram (diagram 1) showing the distribution of rats in both populations we can observe greater concentrations around the average figure in rats treated with 7 C Arsenicum Album (maximum difference: 9.60 – 8.65 = 0.95 g) whereas rats treated with 7 C Potentized Water display higher than the average blood concentrations with a maximum difference of 1.69 µg.

Diagram 1

Diagram showing the distribution of rats according to the classification of their blood concentrations into the defined categories:

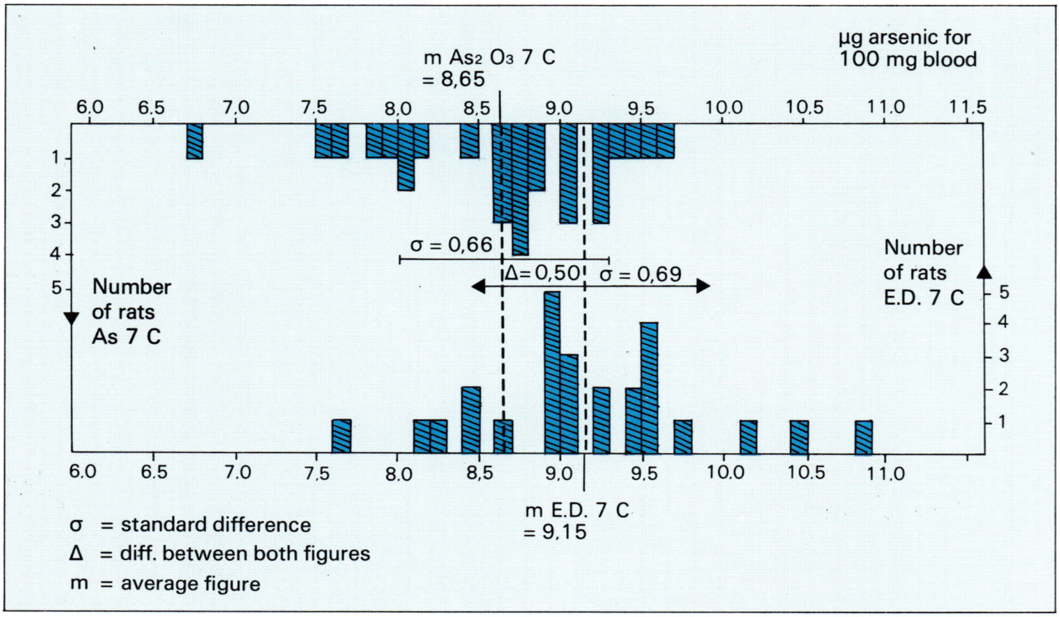

2. WITH ELIMINATION

The increased elimination of arsenic (Charts II and III, Diagrams 2 and 3) during the period of time (12 to 20 h) following its administration in rats treated with a 7 C Arsenicum Album Hahnemanian potency injected at To + 12 h is in accordance with results to be observed in blood: rats treated with 7 C Potentized Water eliminate 13.78 µg arsenic within the 8 hours (To + 20 h) following the administration of the Hahnemanian potency; this, for rats treated with a 7 C Arsenicum Album potency means a 60% increase of arsenious elimination as compared to rats treated with 7 C Potentized Water. THIS DIFFERENCE between 2 batches of 30 rats having the same treatment IS SIGNIFICANT WITH an accuracy rate of 99% (this statistical significance was obtained from Fisher-Snedecor and Student tests).

Chart II

Blood, urine and feces concentrations of arsenic			
Concentrations (µg As/100 mg) measured in: / Batch of 30 rats treated with:	**7 C Arsenicum album**	**7 C Potentized water**	**S.I.**
Blood	8.65 ± 0.66	9.15 ± 0.69	+++
Urine	0.09 ± 0.21	0.07 ± 0.21	●
Feces	1.12 ± 0.21	0.89 ± 0.21	++++

S.I.: Statistical Interpretation (Student's law after analyzing the results):

● : *difference significant above 80 %*
●● : *difference significant above 90 %*
+ : *difference significant above 95 %*
++ : *difference significant above 98 %*
+++ : *difference significant above 99 %*
++++ : *difference significant above 99.9 %*

Diagram 2

Representation of arsenic concentrations, measured in blood, urine and feces of 30 rats treated with 7 C Arsenicum Album and of 30 rats treated with 7 C Potentized Water on semi-logarithmic scale

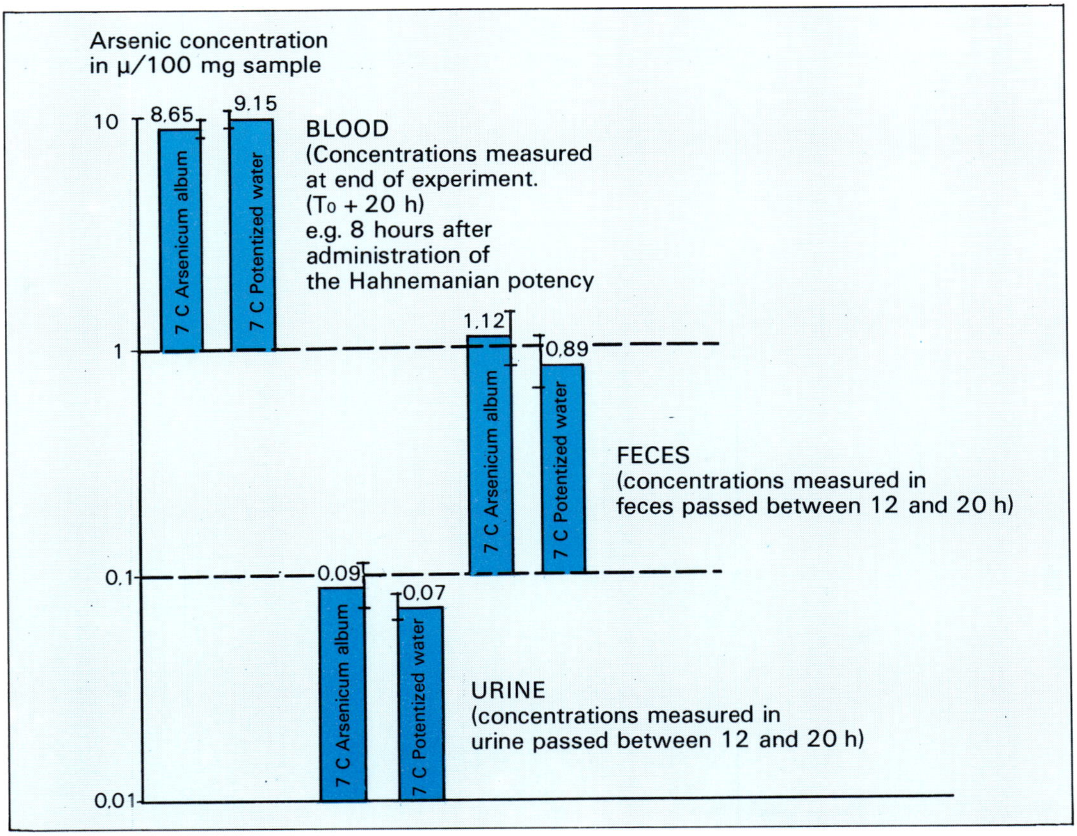

Chart III

Elimination of arsenic in urine and feces			
Batch of 30 rats treated with: / Elimination in µg As per rat	**7 C Arsenicum album**	**7 C Potentized water**	**S.I.**
Feces	20.76 ± 3.52	13.01 ± 3.07	++++
Urine	1.22 ± 0.32	0.77 ± 0.10	++++
Urine + Feces	21.98 ± 3.84	13.78 ± 3.17	++++

S.I.: Statistical Interpretation - see Chart II.

Diagram 3

Elimination of Arsenic during the period of time (T_0 + 12 h to T_0 + 20 h)

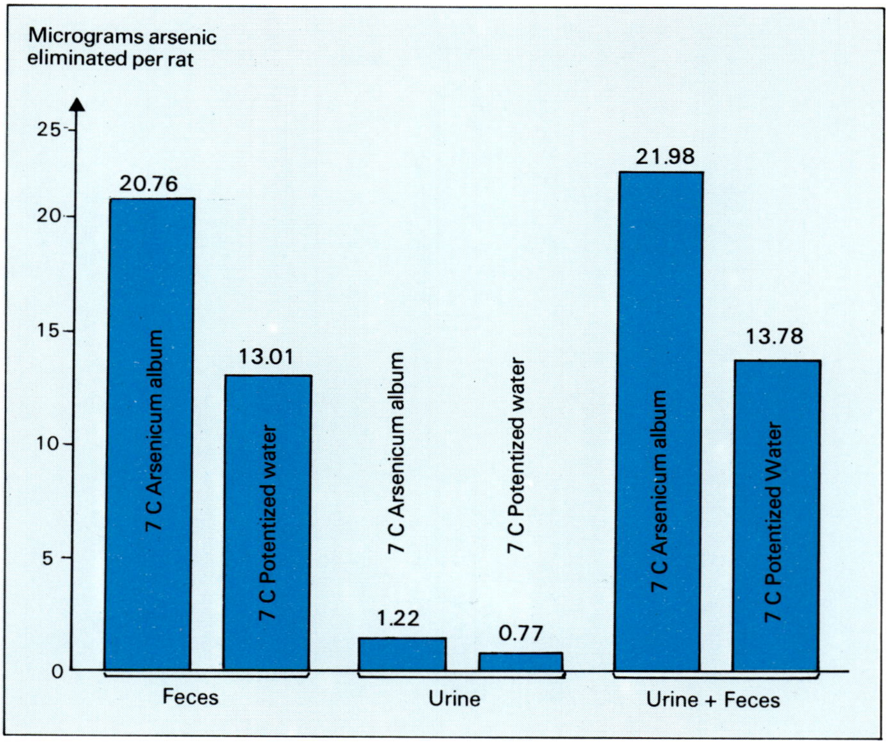

CONCLUSION

ONE SINGLE 1 ML INJECTION of a Hahnemanian potency of 7 C Arsenicum Album injected intraperitoneally, 12 hours after the per os administration of the toxic solution ENABLED THE 30 RATS TREATED IN THIS WAY TO ELIMINATE 60% MORE ARSENIC in an 8 hour period following the injection than the 30 rats treated in the same way with a 7 C potency of Potentized Water.

THIS DEMONSTRATES THAT A SIGNIFICANT DIFFERENCE EXISTS between both populations of 30 rats, such difference being in favor of the rats treated with 7 C Arsenicum Album with an accuracy rate of 99% (Diagram A).

Diagram A

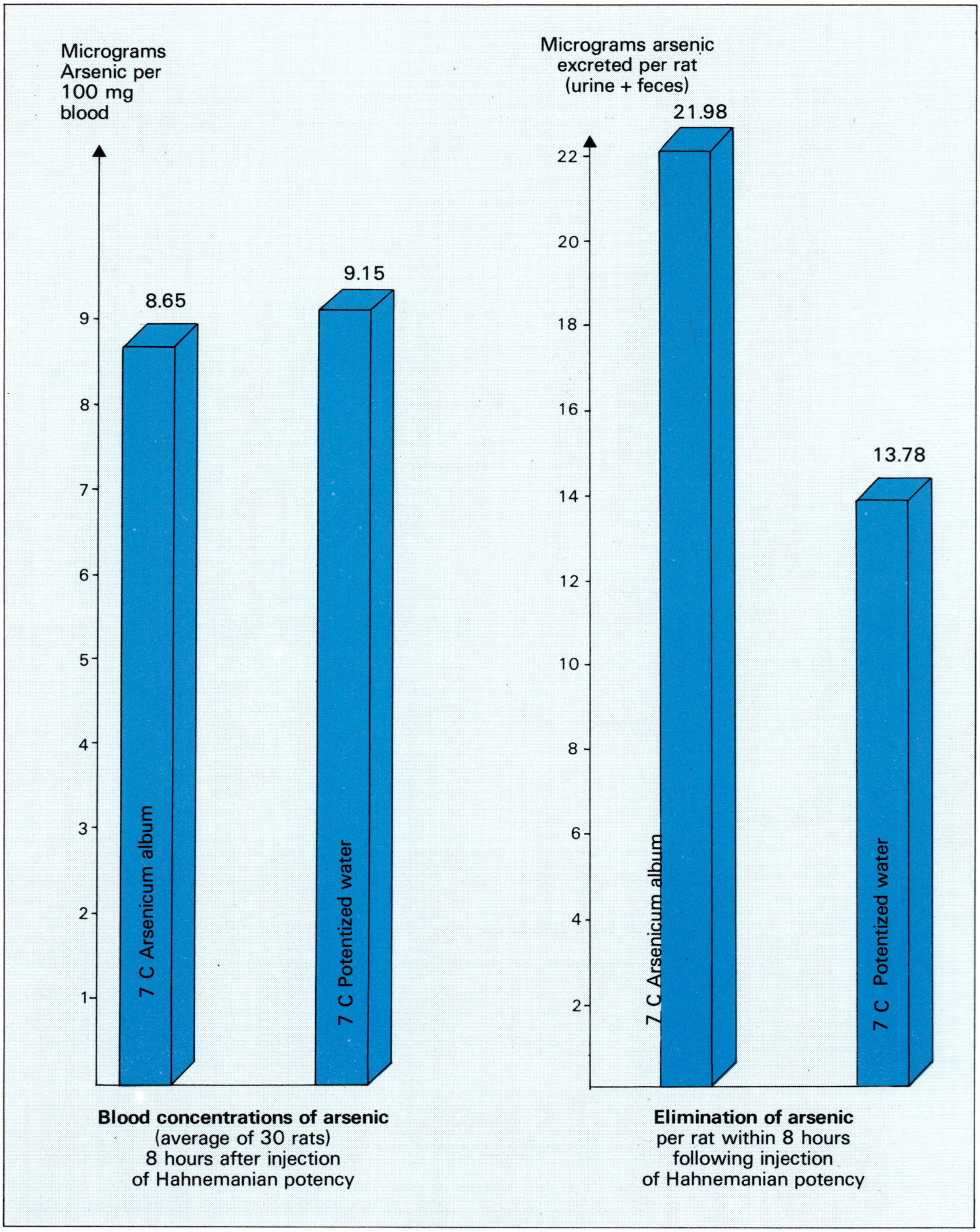

Diagrams showing differences measured in rats treated with 7 C Arsenicum Album on one hand, and in rats treated with 7 C Potentized Water on the other hand (1 ml intraperitoneally). 12 hours after administration of As_2O_3 (irradiated with ^{73}As).

Second test in vivo: effect of three injections of Hahnemanian solutions

MATERIAL AND METHODS

Fifty rats were given per os at To the toxic solution of radio-active arsenic, in the same way and in the same doses as in the first experiment.

Twelve hours later (To + 12 h) we administered intraperitoneally 1 ml of a 7 C Hahnemanian potency of Arsenicum Album to 25 rats taken at random, and 1 ml of 7 C Potentized Water to the last 25 ones under the same conditions.

We performed a second injection at To + 24 h, and a final one at To + 36 h. At To + 7 days, a sample of blood was taken from each rat. All along these 7 days, arsenic elimination was measured.

ANALYZED RESULTS

1. WITH BLOOD

BLOOD CONCENTRATIONS IN ARSENIC for the 25 rats treated with 3 injections of 1 ml 7 C Arsenicum Album ARE, ON AN AVERAGE, LOWER THAN AVERAGE CONCENTRATIONS IN RATS TREATED WITH 7 C POTENTIZED WATER (Chart IV).

- 7 C Arsenicum Album average: 6.27 µg/100 mg blood.
- 7 C Potentized Water average: 6.91 µg/100 mg blood.

The difference of 0.64 µg existing between both batches of 25 rats is significant according to the Fisher-Snedecor and Student tests, with an accuracy rate of 99%.

A study of the diagram showing the classification of rats according to their blood concentrations in Arsenic ranking 0.1 µg per 0.1 µg (chart IV) displays the fact that, OUT OF THE 25 RATS TREATED WITH 7 C ARSENICUM ALBUM, 23 EVIDENCE BLOOD CONCENTRATIONS LOWER THAN THE AVERAGE BLOOD CONCENTRATIONS OF RATS TREATED WITH 7 C POTENTIZED WATER.

The two batches of rats, which have a closely related classification, appear at slightly different positions on the Arsenic blood concentration scale, this being in favor of rats treated with 7 C Arsenicum Album.

Chart IV

Blood concentrations as measured 7 days after administration of arsenic per os
(results in µg of arsenic for 100 mg blood)

7 C Arsenicum album

– 7.17	– 7.03	– 6.80	– 6.86	– 6.76	– 6.79
– 6.50	– 6.53	– 6.57	– 6.41	– 6.43	– 6.49
– 6.31	– 6.34	– 6.21	– 6.16	– 6.18	– 6.00
– 6.05	– 5.96	– 5.99	– 5.79	– 5.61	– 5.53
– 4.34					

General average = 6.27 ± 0.58

7 C Potentized water

– 9.13	– 8.31	– 8.33	– 7.58	– 7.50	– 7.30
– 7.20	– 7.10	– 7.16	– 7.03	– 6.96	– 6.19
– 6.70	– 6.71	– 6.73	– 6.77	– 6.66	– 5.97
– 6.54	– 6.44	– 6.35	– 6.26	– 6.10	– 5.99
– 6.12					

General average = 6.91 ± 0.78

Diagram 4

Diagram showing the classificationof rats according to their blood concentrations (µ As/100 mg blood), 7 days after the administration of arsenic per os.
(Rats treated with Hahnemanian potencies at To + 12 h., To + 24 h., To + 36 h.)

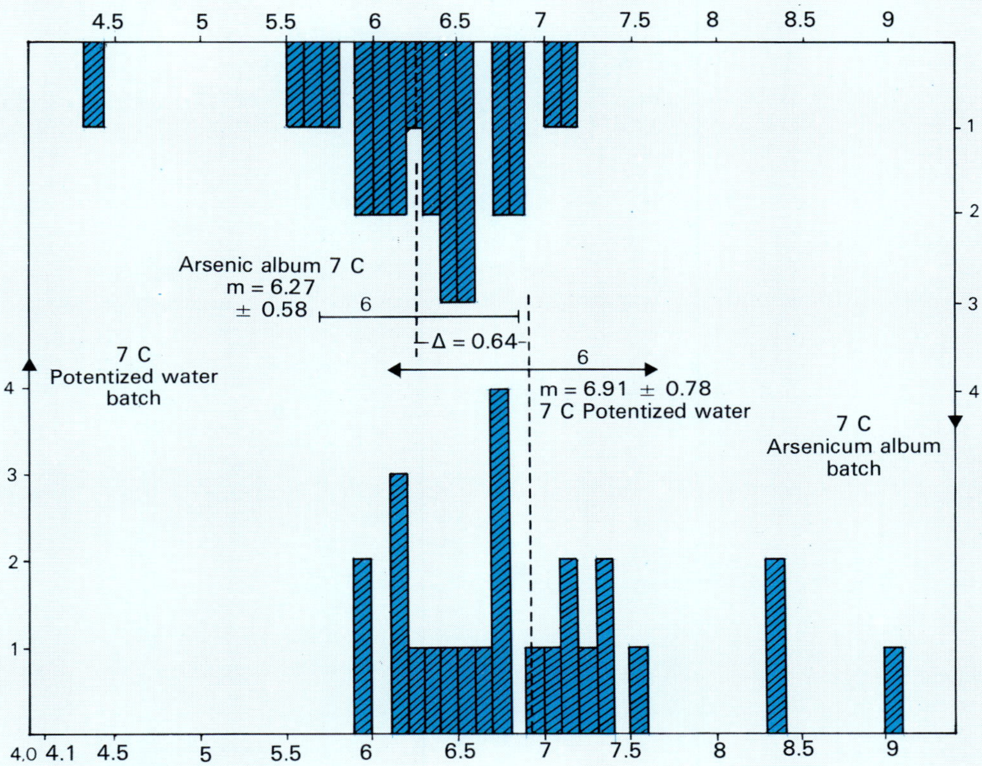

6 = standard difference
Δ = diference between both average figures
m = average figure

2. WITH ELIMINATION

a) In the urine

After two injections have been performed between To and To + 36 h., an increase of URINARY ELIMINATION of arsenic in rats treated with 7 C Arsenicum Album, as compared to rats treated with 7 C Potentized Water can be observed. The rate of this increase AMOUNTS TO 57% FOR 24 HOURS.

AFTER THREE SUCCESSIVE INJECTIONS within the following 36 hours (between To + 36 h. and To + 72 h.) elimination will increase by 44%.

These percentages display significant differences (Fisher-Snedecor and Student tests), with an accuracy rate of 99.9%.

Beyond To + 72 h., the amounts of arsenic eliminated by the two batches are too slight not to diminish the significance of a comparison between them, however, rats treated with 7 C Arsenicum Album will eliminate 80% more arsenic in 24 hours than rats treated with 7 C Potentized Water under the same conditions.

Chart V

Elimination of arsenic in the urine in µg per rat					
Urine passed between	7 C arsenicum album	7 C potentized water	Statistical Analysis		
			Δ	significance	Δ+ in %
12 h - 36 h	4.59 ± 1.42	2.92 ± 0.38	1.67	++++	57.2
36 h - 72 h	3.75 ± 0.34	2.61 ± 0.75	1.14	++++	43.7
72 h - 96 h	0.45 ± 0.28	0.25 ± 0.24	0.20	+++	80

Δ : difference between 7 C Arsenicum album and 7 C Potentized water batches
Significant difference with an accuracy rate of
++++ : ⩾ 99.9 %
+++ : ⩾ 99 %
Δ+ in % : % arsenic eliminated in addition by rats treated with 7 C Arsenicum album

Diagram 5

Elimination of arsenic in the urine

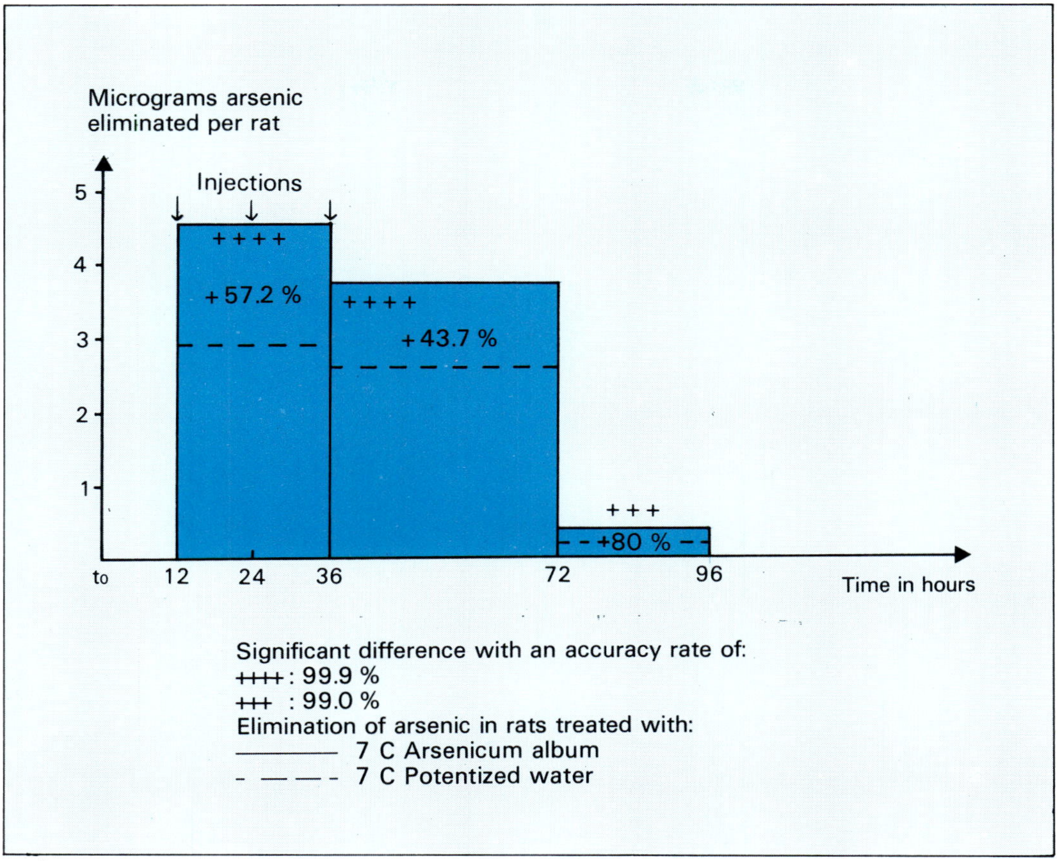

Chart VI

Elimination of arsenic in the urine (in µg per rat - cumulative values)					
Cumulative values over	**7 C Arsenicum album**	**7 C Potentized water**	**Statistical analysis**		
			Δ	significance	Δ+ in %
12 h - 36 h	4.59 ± 1.42	2.92 ± 0.88	1.67	++++	57.2
12 h - 72 h	8.34 ± 1.76	5.53 ± 1.63	2.81	++++	50.8
12 h - 96 h	8.79 ± 2.04	5.78 ± 1.87	3.01	++++	52.1

Δ : difference between 7 C Arsenicum album and 7 C Potentized water batches
Significant difference with an accuracy rate of :
++++ : 99.9 %
Δ+ in % : % arsenic eliminated in addition by rats treated with 7 C Arsenicum album

Diagram 6

Elimination of Arsenic in the urine (cumulative values)

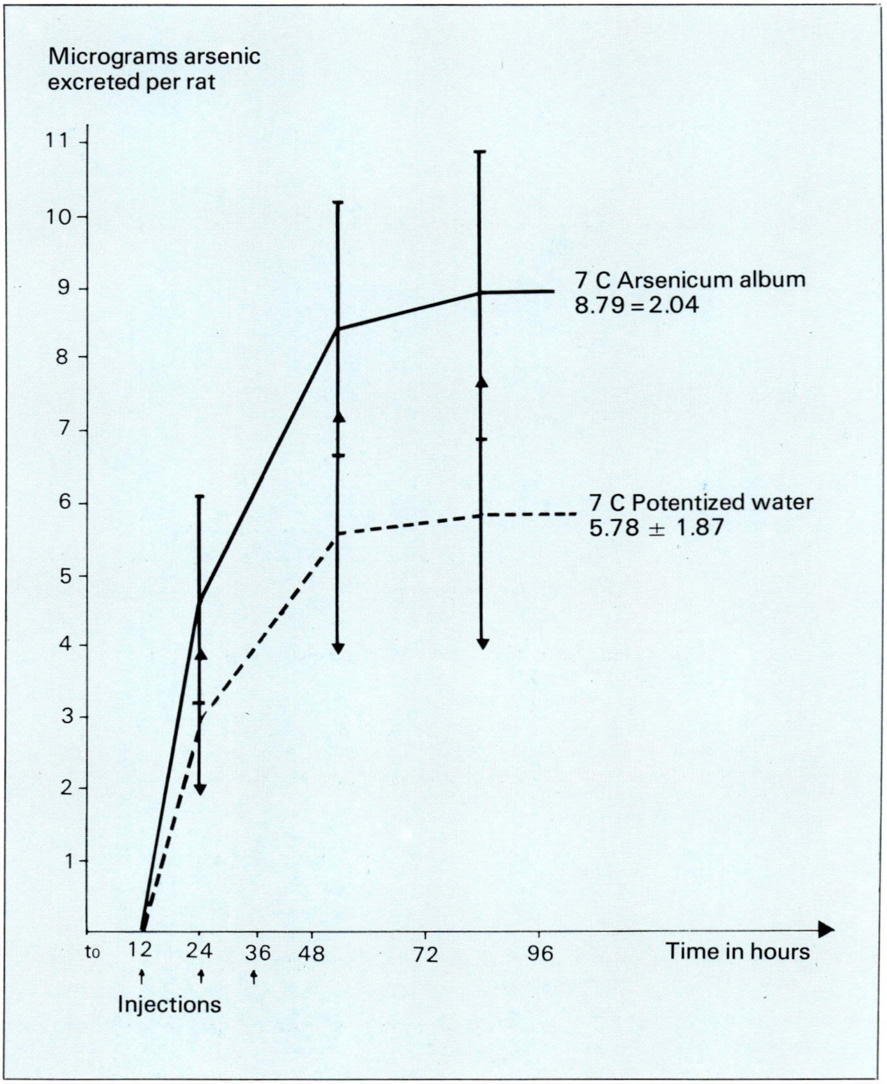

b) In the feces

Rats having received two injections of 7 C Arsenicum Album between To and To + 24 h. eliminate in the feces TWICE AS MUCH arsenic as rats treated with 7 C Potentized Water.

Afterwards, and up to 96 h, elimination decreases and becomes stabilized (Chart 7, Diagram 7).

Tableau VII

Elimination of arsenic (in the feces (in µg per rat - cumulative values)					
Cumulative values over	7 C Arsenicum album	7 C Potentized water	Statistical analysis		Δ^+ in %
			Δ	significance	
12 h - 36 h	79.04 ± 19.57	43.20 ± 15.59	35.84	++++	83.0
12 h - 72 h	82.66 ± 20.82	47.69 ± 17.07	34.97	++++	73.3
12 h - 96 h	85.59 ± 21.50	50.50 ± 17.70	35.09	++++	69.5

Δ *: difference between 7 C Arsenicum album and 7 C Potentized water batches*
Significant difference with an accuracy rate of :
++++ *: 99.9 %*
Δ^+ *in % : % arsenic eliminated in addition by rats treated with 7 C Arsenicum album*

Diagram 7

Elimination of arsenic in the feces (in µg) (cumulative values)

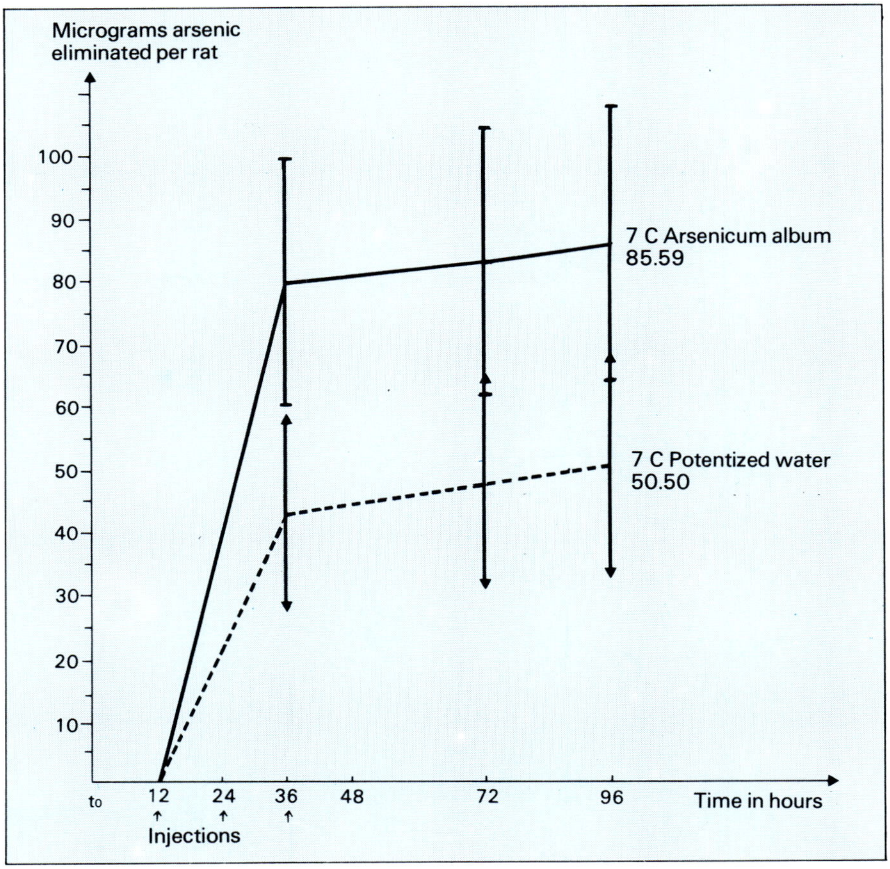

c) Cumulative elimination, in urine and feces

The sum-total of arsenic elimination, both in urine and feces, (Chart 8 - Diagram 8) demonstrates

– that a rat treated 3 times with 1 ml 7 C Arsenicum Album eliminates 95 µg arsenic from 12 h to 96 h,

– that a rat treated 3 times with 1 ml 7 C Potentized Water eliminates 57 µg arsenic during the same period of time.

The difference, e.g 38 µg is significant and evidences a 68% increase of the elimination of arsenic in rats treated with 7 C Arsenicum Album as compared to rats treated with 7 C Potentized Water.

Chart VIII

Elimination of arsenic in urine + feces in µg per rat					
Cumulative values over	7 C Arsenicum album	7 C Potentized water	Statistical analysis		
			Δ	significance	Δ^+ in %
12 h - 36 h	83.63 ± 20.99	46.12 ± 16.47	37.51	++++	81.3
12 h - 72 h	91.00 ± 22.58	53.22 ± 18.70	37.78	++++	71.0
12 h - 96 h	94.38 ± 23.53	56.28 ± 19.57	38.10	++++	67.7

Δ : difference between 7 C Arsenicum album and 7 C Potentized water batches
Significant difference with an accuracy rate of :
++++ : 99.9 %
Δ^+ in % : % arsenic eliminated in addition by rats treated with 7 C Arsenicum album

Diagram 8

Elimination of arsenic in both urine + feces (cumulative values)

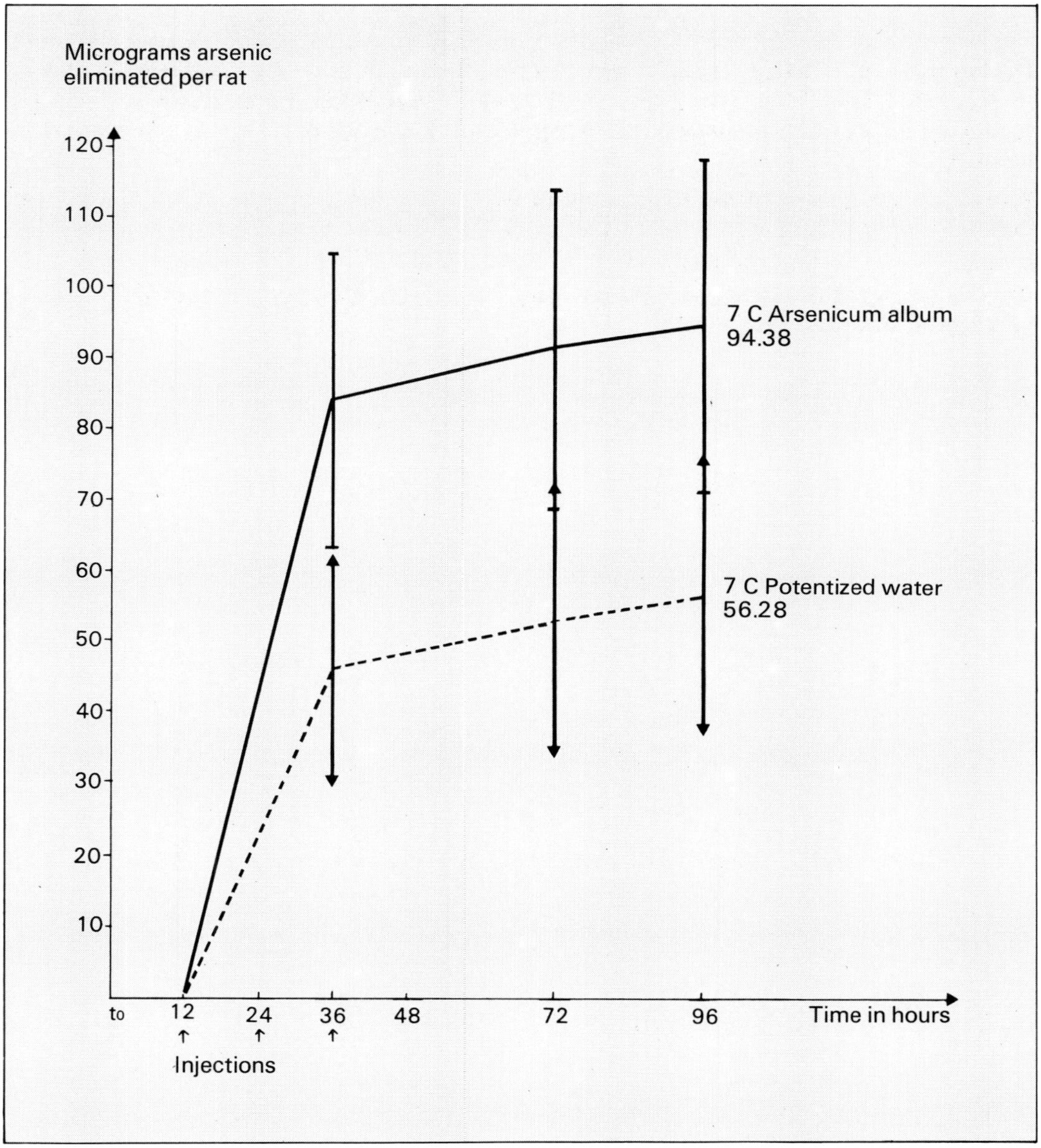

CONCLUSION

During this test in which we administered Hahnemanian potencies in three injections, at To + 12 h., To + 24 h., To + 36 h., we observed, 7 days after the administration of the toxic solution of radio-active arsenic, a significant difference of blood concentrations in arsenic.

Blood concentrations of the batch treated with 7 C Arsenicum Album are lower than blood concentrations of the batch treated with 7 C Potentized Water; elimination of arsenic is clearly superior in the first batch as compared with the second batch.

Results show that the first two injections are responsible for the major part of the observed effect. (Diagram B).

Diagram B

Compared blood concentrations and eliminations

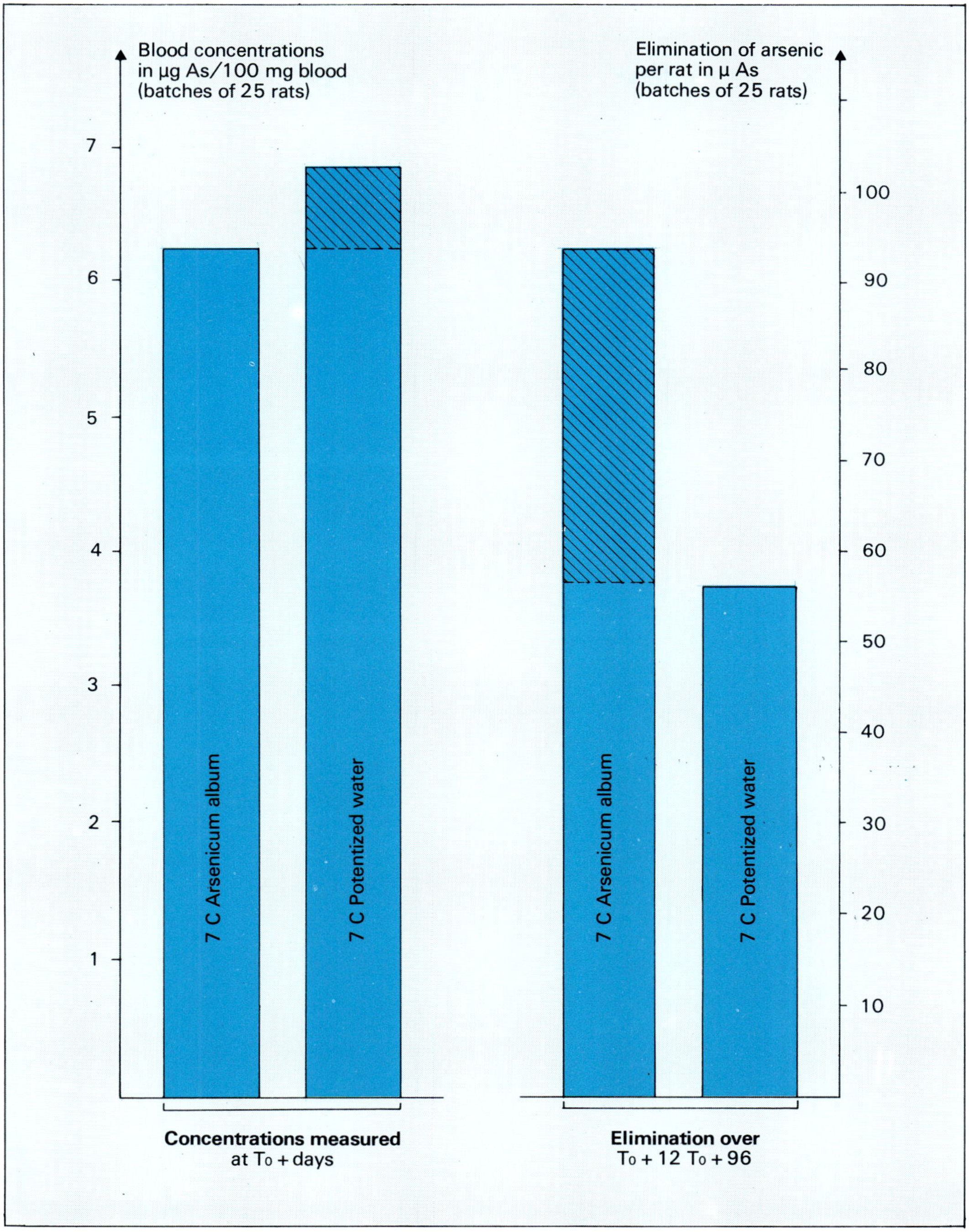

Diagram showing the differences measured between a) rats treated with 7 C Arsenicum album and b) rats treated with 7 C Potentized water after the administration of As_2O_3 (irradiated by ^{73}As).

SECTION III

THE ACTION OF GELSEMIUM SEMPERVIRENS TINCTURE UPON THE CAPTURE OF NEUROTRANSMITTERS BY SYNAPTOSOMAL PREPARATIONS OF VARIOUS FRACTIONS OF RAT BRAIN

INTRODUCTION

GELSEMIUM SEMPERVIRENS – Jasmium Virginianum – is an extremely poisonous plant. Its use in Homeopathy is indicated notably in the treatment of stage-fright, particularly when it is accompanied by obsession, temporary loss of memory, or a tendency to diarrhea.

Poisoning by this vegetable substance produces a two-phase reaction in the cerebrospinal system : during the first phase, the patient quivers, has cramps, and coordination problems. In the second phase, paresis appears, caused by passive congestion of the brain and medulla.

Thanks to the psychopharmacological research work performed by Laborit* in 1952 on the therapeutic effects of chlorpromazine, it is known that the action of this tranquilizer corresponds to an increase in the metabolites of certain neuro-transmitters. Thus, an increase in dopamine metabolites under the effect of chlorpromazine was evidenced in 1965. Subsequently, thanks to the work of Cooper* (1978) Hall and Hildebrand* (1974), Iversen and Bird* (1979-1980), it clearly appeared that the pharmacological action of neuroleptics could have an effect at the neuro-transmitters capturing level besides other channels.

The model most generally accepted for describing the transmission of nerve impulse is the following: the transmission of the nerve impulse from one neuron to another within the synapsis takes place through the liberation of a chemical mediator fixing itself onto a post-synaptic receptor, thus inducing a new potential.

The main way of inactivating the mediator liberated in the synaptic space is a re-absorption of the contents of the pre-synaptic vesicle previously liberated (called "capture").

This "capture" of the neurotransmitter (or mediator) through the synaptic membrane, active phenomenon (Henn* in 1971), ouabaïne-sensitive (Baldessarini* in 1973) Nak dependent (Bruinvels* in 1975) constitutes the main way of inactivating the neuro-transmitter which has been liberated within the intersynaptic space.

This "capture" phenomenon depends on temperature and requires the presence of A.T.P. (Adenosine-triphosphate) (Schwartz* in 1971).

The "in vivo" study of such capture is difficult to perform (Nioulhon* in 1977), however "in vitro" techniques have been developed, using, for instance, either sections (Shaskan* in 1970) or homogenates (Snyder* in 1969), and are reliable models of phenomena existing "in vivo". Indeed, when nerve cells are destroyed through crushing, the nerve-endings will form new vesicles, known as synaptosomes, endowed with some of the properties of the intact neuron (Snyder* in 1969).

The parallelism which exists between the indications of certain neuroleptics and the use made of Gelsemium in Homeopathy led us to study the effect of Gelsemium tincture and its potencies upon the capture of various neuro-transmitters: noradrenalin (NA), dopamine (DA) and serotonine (5 HT) by synaptosomal preparations of various fractions of brain tissue.

---

* See bibliography.

MATERIAL AND METHODS

1. CAPTURE OF NEURO-TRANSMITTERS BY RAT SYNAPTOSOMES HAVING RECEIVED NO PREVIOUS TREATMENT

a) Mode of operation

The rats (males of a Wistar strain, weighing 180-250 g), were decapitated and the brain was quickly dissected into five parts:

- brainstem;
- mesencephalon;
- hypothalamus;
- corpus striatum;
- cortex.

Before dissection was performed, brains were rinsed with NaCl 0.9%. The section to be studied was set in 0.32 M saccharose (weight of the cerebral section/weight of the saccharose solution = 1 to 4). It was then crushed in a Potter device (Thomas B 55-20%), until a homogeneous suspension was obtained.

The homogenate was then centrifuged at 1 000 g for 10 mn. The deposit containing cell fragments was eliminated. The supernatant liquid contained the synaptosomes, which should be kept in appropriate media if their properties are to be maintained.

A Krebs Henselheit medium was used here. This medium was oxygenated for 10 minutes by use of a carbogenic mixture (O_2: 95% and CO_2: 5%) the Ph of which is 7.2-7.3 when measured cold.

The Gelsemium tincture was then added to this Krebs medium to the 1/10th (Gelsemium sempervirens TE 0862 - Laboratoires Boiron).

During these tests, 0.3 ml of brain homogenate was added to 3 ml of Krebs medium.

After a pre-incubation period of 5 mn at a temperature of 37° C in a double-boiler equipped with an agitator, the tritium irradiated mediator was added (0.2 ml of a 17.5 10^{-7} solution was added. These 0.2 ml had a radio-activity of 0.1 μCi). Incubation was maintained for 5 mn.

Capture was stopped by shaking the tubes in soft ice. These tubes were then centrifuged for 15 mn at 25 000 gr. The supernatant was eliminated.

The deposit containing the synaptosomes was drained and rinsed with 3 ml ice-cold NaCl 0.9%. In order to obtain an accurate evaluation of the radio-activity, it was then homogenized by adding 2 ml of iced absolute alcohol with a strong agitation in the cyclo-mixer, for the first series of tests. Replacement of alcohol by Krebs for the second series of tests ensured a better homogeneous suspension.

The amount of tritiated mediator contained in the synaptosomes was then evaluated after the addition of 10 ml of a scintillating solution (Rac Gel 33) in a liquid scintillation counter (Packard). An average of at least two counts was calculated.

"Blanks", identical to each kind of trials underwent a same treatment but were kept in soft ice. The capture of the mediator was defined by the difference existing between the radioactivity measured in the trials and the one contained in the blanks.

The essays were quadrupled, each figure being the average of four determinations.

b) Selection of experimental conditions

Conditions for capture are very strict.

TEMPERATURE

37° C was selected as it corresponds to optimal conditions for the enzymatic system (at a lower temperature the rate of reaction speed is lesser: high temperatures cause denaturation.

TIME

Capture value is proportional to time. For the time selected here, (relatively short: 5 mn after introduction of the radioactive mediator), release is sufficiently weak so as not to interfere with measures.

CONCENTRATION OF MEDIATOR

This concentration is of 10^{-7}; with this concentration, a high affinity capture (Km = 10^{-7} M) and the participation of the low affinity system (Km 10^{-4} to 10^{-6}) is negligible.

In order to obtain this 10^{-7} M concentration in the case of the 5 HT, the 5 HT with a specific activity of 500 mCi/mM supplied (like DA and NA) by the French Atomic Energy Commission was soluted directly in the Krebs.

NA 10^7 was obtained by mixing NA 10^3M preserved in a frozen state, and then diluted, with tritiated NA (specific activity 4.5 Ci/mM).

The same applies for DA (specific activity of tritiated DA: 18 Ci/mM).

CONCENTRATION OF THE BRAIN HOMOGENATE

It was precisely determined by performing a quantitative analysis of proteins (Biuret method according to Gornall*) in order to be able to express the capture per mg of proteins, so as to compare the various experiments.

- for a study of the cortex, 3 rat brains were used;
- for a study of the brainstem, 4 rat brains were used;
- for a study of the mesencephalon, 4 rat brains were used;
- for a study of the corpus striatum, 9 rat brains were used;
- for a study of the hypothalamus, 9 rat brains were used.

These brains were crushed in saccharose 0.32 M (one part brain for four parts saccharose).

CONCENTRATION OF THE DRUG

In a first series of experiments, Gelsemium tincture was studied in final concentration in trials with 10^{-2}, 10^{-4}, 10^{-7}, 10^{-10}. Results were compared to those obtained with control solutions containing only the brain-Krebs and the mediator, and with control solutions of an identical composition although containing alcohol in the same concentration as in the tincture, in case such alcohol would have a possible effect upon the capture.

The quantity of tincture having to be contained in the 3 ml of Krebs introduced in this trial was calculated by taking account of the final volume (3.5 ml) after the brain homogenate and the mediator were added.

The solution with a final concentration of 10^{-2} of tincture in the trial contained: 1.2 ml of Gelsemium tincture + 98.8 ml of Krebs (solution A).

The solution with a final concentration of 10^{-4} contained: 1 ml solution A + 99.ml Krebs (solution B).

The solution with a final concentration of 10^{-7} contained: 0.1 ml of solution B + 99.9 ml of Krebs (solution C).

The solution with a final concentration of 10^{-10} contained: 0.1 ml of solution C + 99.9 ml of Krebs.

The different solutions which were contained in identical vessels were then agitated, so that the disappearance of oxygen caused by agitating the Krebs might remain approximately the same. For the alcohol control solutions, the Krebs used contained: 1.2 ml absolute alcohol + 98.8 ml of Krebs, which corresponds to an addition of 36 µl in the trial.

In the second series of trials, a few alterations were made so as to operate under stricter conditions.

- Vessels were not cleaned with HCl. They were rinsed in water several times, and then again with filtered water. A same vessel was always used for a same concentration of the drug.
- Weaker concentrations of Gelsemium tincture (10^{-14}, 10^{-18}) were tried. In order that tests performed remain comparable to those of the first series, trials were carried out with 10^{-2} and 10^{-10} tinctures (final concentrations always used in trials), and this for each of the alcohol control-solutions. Trials were reproduced four times.

POTENCIES

The mode of operation used was always the same, as follows:

Potencies were made on the morning of the test with 61% alcohol (this titration corresponding to the titration of the tincture), such titration of alcohol being obtained by agitating a mixture of pure alcohol and distilled water kept in a glass container, for 15 minutes.

Solution D = 0.120 ml Gelsemium tincture + 9.88 ml alcohol (sol. $1.2.10^{-2}$).

Solution E = 0.100 ml sol. A + 9.90 ml alcohol (sol.$1.2.10^{-4}$).

Solution F = 0.100 ml sol. B + 9.90 ml alcohol (sol.$1.2.10^{-6}$).

Solution G + 0.100 ml sol. C + 9.90 ml alcohol (Sol.$1.2.10^{-8}$).

The $1.2.10^{-16}$ was reached by degrees, through all intermediate stages, (10^{-10}, 10^{-12}, 10^{-14}).

In identical Erlenmayer flasks, each containing 99 ml oxygenated Krebs medium (98.8 ml in the case of 10^{-2}) the following were added:

- 1.2 ml of Gelsemium tincture to obtain a final 10^{-2} for the trial;
- 1 ml of the 10^{-8} alcohol-tincture mixture (sol.D) to obtain a final 10^{-10};
- 1 ml of the 10^{-12} alcohol-tincture mixture to obtain a final 10^{-14};
- 1 ml of the 10^{-16} alcohol-tincture mixture to obtain a final 10^{-18}.

AGITATION

The 10 ml tubes were agitated at full speed in a cyclo-mixer for at least 5 seconds.

The Erlenmayer flasks containing 100 ml were agitated for at least 5 minutes.

All these reagents were kept in soft ice.

The work was performed as quickly as possible after rats' decapitation, in order that brain homogenate activity be maintained for a maximum period of time.

2. CAPTURE OF NEUROTRANSMITTERS BY SYNAPTOSOMES OF UNSTRESSED RATS TREATED IN VIVO WITH GELSEMIUM TINCTURE

a) Case of a single injection

These tests were carried out upon 6 male rats of same weight and same age, having received a single injection of Gelsemium tincture (20 µl in 1 ml isotonic NaCl 0.9% - while 6 control rats received only 1 ml NaCl 0.9%).

The animals were decapitated 24 hours after being injected. The brains were quickly removed and dissected. The homogenates corresponding to the different parts of the brain were stored at a low temperature. Each batch of 6 rats was in turn divided into 3 batches of 2 animals each.

Tubes corresponding to each batch of control-rats were intercalated among those corresponding to the treated rats. The trials were reproduced four times for each batch.

The mode of operation was kept the same as in the preceding test, and the average of the 3 "captures" in treated rats was compared to the 3 "captures" in control rats.

Three mediators were used: NA, DA, 5 HT, with parts of the brain having a special affinity for each of them, as done in the previous test.

The following were studied:

1) NA with mesencephalon.

2) 5 HT with brainstem.

3) DA with corpus striatum.

b) Case of 15 injections (20 µl at each time)

Identical tests were performed with rats of a same age and weight. For 15 days in succession, they received an intra-peritoneal injection of Gelsemium tincture (20 µl in 1 ml NaCl 0.9%).

6 control rats were placed in similar conditions and also received a daily injection of NaCl 0.9% for 15 days.

Both control and drugged rats weighed the same weight at the end of the 15 days.

They were sacrificed 24 hours after the last injection.

The following elements were studied:

1) NA with mesencephalon.

2) 5 HT with brainstem.

3) 5 HT with hypothalamus.

ANALYZED RESULTS

1. TESTS PERFORMED UPON HOMOGENATES OF UNTREATED RAT BRAINS

a) A study of NA capture (Chart 1)

10^{-2} CONCENTRATION

At a concentration of 10^{-2}, Gelsemium tincture causes a strong inhibition (above 50%) which is more or less significant depending on the part of brain being studied. It is very marked with brainstem (85% in the first series of tests and nearly total in the second).

Chart I

NA Capture								
Level / Concentration	Cortex		Brain stem		Mesencephalon		Hypothalamus	
	Test 1	Test 2	Test 1	Test 2	Test 1	Test 2	Test 1	Test 2
10^{-2}	52	28	15	0	51	27	40	15
Relative uncertainty %	± 0.8 %	± 11.2 %	± 16 %	± 2.72 %	± 4 %	± 3.31 %	± 5 %	± 1.92 %
10^{-4}	86	–	76	–	79	–	100	–
Relative uncertainty %	± 6 %	–	± 8 %	–	± 10 %	–	± 5 %	–
10^{-7}	88	–	98	–	90	–	105	–
Relative uncertainty %	± 8 %	–	± 3 %	–	± 7.6 %	–	± 3 %	–
10^{-10}	94	116	107	103	90	121	110	110
Relative uncertainty %	± 4 %	± 3.78 %	± 2 %	± 6.54 %	± 3.4 %	± 2.04 %	± 2 %	± 1.6 %
10^{-14}	–	93	–	105	–	107	–	99.4
Relative uncertainty %	–	± 2.55 %	–	± 4.2 %	–	± 3.98 %	–	± 1.7 %
10^{-18}	–	99	–	80	–	112	–	105
Relative uncertainty %	–	± 3.3 %	–	± 2.71 %	–	± 4.12 %	–	± 1.6 %

(The 100 % value corresponds here to NA capture in untreated control subjects)

10^{-4} CONCENTRATION

At a concentration of 10^{-4}, the inhibition subsists, however at a lesser degree.

10^{-7} CONCENTRATION

In the case of a 10^{-7} concentration inhibition is even weaker; there might even be a reverse phenomena in some cases. A slight activation of approximately 5% is observed in the case of hypothalamus.

10^{-10} CONCENTRATION

In the case of a 10^{-10} concentration, there seems to be a slight increase in "capture" in the case of cortex (16% for the second series only) and a very slight increase for brainstem (in both series). An increase was also observed for mesencephalon (second series only). For hypothalamus a 10% activation is observed (identical figures in both series).

A test conducted with 15 tubes containing tincture and 15 control tubes set in contact with mesencephalon homogenate + hypothalamus confirms that a slight increase of "capture" takes place.

10^{-14} CONCENTRATION

In the case of a 10^{-14} concentration, there is practically no action, except, perhaps, a very slight activation for mesencephalon.

10^{-18} CONCENTRATION

A 10^{-18} concentration seems to have no effect, except, perhaps, a slight increase for mesencephalon and a slight inhibition for brainstem.

b) A study of DA capture (Chart 2)

10^{-2} CONCENTRATION

In the case of a 10^{-2} concentration, inhibition is very strong, and is identical for both series (70% for cortex and 80% at least for corpus striatum).

10^{-4} CONCENTRATION

Inhibition is approximately 30% for corpus striatum. It is slightly weaker for cortex.

10^{-7} CONCENTRATION

In the case of a 10^{-7} concentration, the rate of "capture" decreases by about 30% for corpus striatum.

Chart II

DA capture

Concentration \ Level	Cortex		Corpus striatum	
	Test 1	Test 2	Test 1	Test 2
10^{-2}	32	6	20	12
Relative uncertainty %	± 2 %	± 1.74 %	± 2 %	± 5.8 %
10^{-4}	76	–	68	–
Relative uncertainty %	± 13 %	–	± 7.9 %	–
10^{-7}	106	–	72	–
Relative uncertainty %	± 5 %	–	± 4 %	–
10^{-10}	125	110	79	96
Relative uncertainty %	± 6 %	± 5.63 %	± 9.4 %	± 2.14 %
10^{-14}	–	117	–	108
Relative uncertainty %	–	± 1.44 %	–	± 8.25 %
10^{-18}	–	102	–	99
Relative uncertainty %	–	± 3.68 %	–	± 2.39 %

10^{-10} CONCENTRATION

In both series of tests a slight inhibition can be observed in the case of corpus striatum. Inversely, in the case of cortex, there is a 25% increase in the first series and a 10% increase in the second series.

10^{-14} CONCENTRATION

A slight increase is evidenced in the case of corpus striatum and a 17% increase for cortex.

10^{-18} CONCENTRATION

This concentration seems to have no action.

c) A study of 5 HT capture (Chart III)

10^{-2} CONCENTRATION

Inhibition is very strong, higher than 50%. It is nearly total for hypothalamus in both series of tests.

10^{-4} CONCENTRATION

Inhibition is about 40% for brainstem and mesencephalon and nearly total for the cortex and the hypothalamus. There might be a very slight activation for corpus striatum.

10^{-7} CONCENTRATION

There is a slight inhibition everywhere except for corpus striatum for which there is in fact a 14% activation.

10^{-10} CONCENTRATION

Activation is slight for the mesencephalon. It is stronger in the case of hypothalamus. It is above 20% in the second series of tests. The test involving 15 tubes with 10^{-10} tincture in the presence of control batches confirms this (see further on).

10^{-14} CONCENTRATION

A 13% activation is to be noted for mesencephalon, together with a very slight inhibition with cortex and brainstem; no action is observed with corpus striatum and hypothalamus.

10^{-18} CONCENTRATION

Very little action is observed, except, perhaps, a slight activation in the case of mesencephalon.

Chart III

5 HT Capture										
Level / Concentration	Cortex		Brainstem		Mesencephalon		Corpus striatum		Hypothalamus	
	Test 1	Test 2	Test 1	Test 2	Test 1	Test 2	Test 1	Test 2	Test 1	Test 2
10^{-2}	54	30	21	4	9	19	16	19	3	6
Relative uncertainty %	± 9 %	± 1.82 %	± 6 %	± 5.84 %	± 11.2 %	± 2.8 %	± 5.8 %	± 0.53 %	± 6 %	± 5.02 %
10^{-4}	93	–	63	–	59	–	104	–	94	–
Relative uncertainty %	± 6.6 %	–	± 2.5 %	–	± 16 %	–	± 2.5 %	–	± 5 %	–
10^{-7}	86	–	83	–	71	–	114	–	87	–
Relative uncertainty %	± 4 %	–	± 3.5 %	–	± 2 %	–	± 1.9 %	–	± 12 %	–
10^{-10}	97	97	82	97	107	105	99	103	112	129
Relative uncertainty %	± 7 %	± 4.23 %	± 7.3 %	± 2.98 %	± 7.3 %	± 3.5 %	± 3 %	± 1.01 %	± 2 %	± 0.81 %
10^{-14}	–	92	–	95	–	113	–	100	–	104
Relative uncertainty %	–	± 4.27 %	–	± 4.58 %	–	± 3.26 %	–	± 3.35 %	–	± 6.62 %
10^{-18}	–	103	–	95	–	115	–	100	–	100
Relative uncertainty %	–	± 1.48 %	–	± 2.73 %	–	± 4.28 %	–	± 5.28 %	–	± 9.7 %

2. TESTS PERFORMED WITH HOMOGENATES OF BRAINS OF RATS TREATED "IN VIVO" WITH GELSEMIUM TINCTURE (Chart 4)

a) Rats having received a single injection of tincture (20 µl)

There seems to be a strong increase in "capture" for all three mediators. This varies according to mediators:

- 55% in the case of NA with mesencephalon;
- 18% in the case of DA with corpus striatum;
- 12% in the case of 5 HT with brainstem.

b) Rats having received 15 injections (of 20 µl of tincture each)

A very strong increase of capture is evidenced here, as in the case of a single injection, as follows:

- 43% in the case of 5 HT with brainstem;
- 28% in the case of NA with mesencephalon.

It only amounts to 2% in the case of 5 HT in the presence of hypothalamus synaptosomes.

Chart IV

Capture of NA in mesencephalon, of 5 HT in brainstem and hypothalamus, of DA in corpus striatum with Gelsemium tincture

	Capture of NA in mesencephal.	Capture of 5 HT in brainstem	Capture of DA in corpus str.	Capture of 5 HT in hypothalamus
Rats having received a single injection of 20 µl of tincture	155 ± 17.80 %	112 ± 30.41 %	118 ± 8.80 %	
Rats having received 15 injections of 20 µl of tincture	128 ± 8.68 %	143 ± 13.93 %		102 ± 23 %

DISCUSSION

We may draw several conclusions from these tests, even though they do deserve some criticism, particularly regarding the following:

In the case of acellular systems, we a priori considered the 1000 g supernatant to be a synaptosomal fraction, knowing that it contains, besides the synaptosomes, microsomes, lysosomes, mitochondrial fragments and the soluble cytoplasmic phase.

We did not intend to obtain a fraction either pure or highly enriched with synaptosomes. We did not think it necessary to control this fraction by use of an electronic microscope, this part of the work being highly standardized and corresponding to previously published operations.

The number of trials carried out, and the number of animals used do not allow for a systematic statistical study. We shall therefore only discuss the results we constantly and ultimately obtained as they reflect significant differences existing between test and control batches.

From results obtained, it was evidenced that Gelsemium tincture at a 10^{-2} concentration causes a very strong inhibition of serotonin, noradrenalin and dopamin captures.

One can reasonably estimate that the active substances account for 0.1 to 3% of the tincture dry weight, the latter making up 1 $\pm$ 0.5% of the total tincture. If molecular weight is around 300, the active substance, the concentration of which is situated between 10^{-5} and 10^{-7} M in our trials, must be one of the drugs able to strongly inhibit the capture.

The activating action of the 10^{-10} concentration is very significant. It is to be found in a number of tests, as new results tend to confirm it. This fact is all the more remarkable that it confirms one of the bases of Homeopathy.

It is to be noted that concentrations causing an activation of the capture of certain neurotransmitters "in vitro" correspond to the 4th and 5th C. Hahnemanian potencies, both of which are widely prescribed by Homeopaths.

At 10^{-4} and 10^{-18} concentrations, the tincture has practically no action upon the model studied.

"In vivo" injections of Gelsemium tincture cause an increase in the capture of neurotransmitters.

This result is highly significant, as it proves the action of the drug injected "in vivo". One might in fact, consider that a drug with an "in vitro" action might have no "in vivo" action, particularly if it was not able to pass the hematomeningeal barriers or if it was rapidly catabolized in the peripheral area.

A more comprehensive study is currently being carried out; it involves a great number of animals and a variety of doses.

Preliminary results confirm that Gelsemium tincture and certain of its potencies has an effect upon the capture of neurotransmitters, hence on nerve impulse.

Nothing prevents us from concluding that the biological mechanism linked to the therapeutical action of this drug may be linked to these phenomena.

SECTION IV

THE EFFECTS OF MERCURIUS CORROSIVUS HAHNEMANIAN POTENCIES UPON THE MULTIPLICATION OF CULTURED FIBROBLASTS POISONED WITH MERCURY CHLORIDE

INTRODUCTION

The favorable effect of Hahnemanian potencies of the toxic agent upon sub-intoxicated systems was evidenced by research work (see Section II) aiming at defining the physiological level at which the therapeutic agent – here the homeopathic potency – is active.

We, consequently, thought it interesting to examine whether it was possible to evidence a possible action of Hahnemanian potencies of this same mercury chloride, i.e. Mercurius corrosivus on fibroblast cultures having been poisoned with the same mercury chloride.

MATERIAL AND METHODS

DETERMINATION OF THE SUB-TOXIC DOSE

The mercury chloride solutions were prepared from a mother-solution of 125 mg for 100 ml distilled water.

Solution 1 : potency at 1/8 of the mother-solution

Solution 2 : potency at 1/9 of the mother-solution

The culture medium was as follows:

- Ham F 10 medium .... 80 ml
- Fetal calf serum .... 20 ml
- Penicillin, 1 million units, + streptomycin 1 g for 10 ml of distilled water .... 0.6 ml
- Fungizone (SQUIBB): solution of 50 mg for 10 ml of distilled water .... 0.4 ml

The fibroblast cultures of human skin were distributed in a series of Corning containers, as shown in Chart I :

Chart I

Determination of the sub-toxic dose of mercury chloride			
	Control	**Test 1**	**Test 2**
Cellular suspension 20,000 elements/ml	1 ml	1 ml	1 ml
Culture medium	1.4 ml	1.4 ml	1.4 ml
Mercury chloride solution 1	0	0.1 ml	0
Mercury chloride solution 2	0	0	0.1 ml
Sterile Distilled Water	0.1 ml	0	0
Concentration in mercury chloride	0	1/160 000	1/180 000

After homogenization was performed, the containers were set in a 37° C stove for 48 hours.

The containers were then removed from the stove and the cells were fixed and colored in the following way:

- after the culture medium was sucked out, 2.5 ml of a hypotonic solution was introduced in the box (fetal calf serum 1 ml, sterile distilled water, 9 ml).
- the containers were set in the 37° C stove for another 10 minutes;
- cell swelling was checked through a microscope;
- one Pasteur pipette of A liquid was then added in small fractions at the four cardinal points (acetic acid, methanol 1/3);
- one Pasteur pipette of B liquid was then added (acetic acid, methanol, distilled water 1/3/4) with a stirring movement near the containers' inner surface; about half a pipette of solution was sucked out;
- this last operation was repeated six times;
- in the same way, and for 8 successive times, one Pasteur pipette of A liquid was then added. However, after each addition, one and a half pipette of supernatant was sucked out;
- when the last operation was completed, the remaining supernatant was sucked out, the container was allowed to air-dry, and coloration was performed with May Grunwald Giemsa;
- a count was then performed under a microscope. 3,000 elements were counted after careful sweeping of the bottom of the container. The mitotic index, in other words, the number of mitosis per 100 cells was calculated.

2. TESTS WITH HAHNEMANIAN POTENCIES

First of all, the cells of a second subculture strain were distributed and treated with Hahnemanian potencies as shown on Chart II after they were collected by trypsination according to the following procedure:

- the culture medium was sucked out. The container was then rinsed twice in a 2.5 ml Puck solution (Puck's saline A (10 x) Gibco 50 ml, Gibco's Bicarbonate of sodium 1 ml, sterile distilled water 400 ml);
- 1 ml trypsin (Gibco's 2.5% trypsin, 10 ml, Puck solution 90 ml) was then added; this was left in contact for one minute, and the supernatant was sucked out until only a thin film of trypsin remained in contact with the cells;
- about 2 ml of the culture medium was then added, and the suspension was homogenized by a successive sucking and blowing out process by means of a Pasteur pipette.

Chart II

Test with Hahnemanian Potencies distributions of components				
	5 C Potentized water control s.	**5 C Mercurius corrosivus**	**15 C Potentized water control s.**	**15 C Mercurius corrosivus**
Cellular suspension 1 million per ml	1 ml	1 ml	1 ml	1 ml
Culture medium	10 ml	10 ml	10 ml	10 ml
5 C Potentized water	0.2 ml	0	0	0
15 C Potentized water	0	0	0.2 ml	0
5 C Mercurius corrosivus	0	0.2 ml	0	0
15 C Mercurius corrosivus	0	0	0	0.2 ml

- flasks were then set in a 37° C stove, and a change of media and of additives was performed on the day after the culture was started.

The operation was repeated twice at 48 hours interval, in order to obtain four additions of the corresponding Hahnemanian potencies, both for control and test solutions.

After seven days, the cells from each flask were collected separately and cell concentration was brought to 20,000 elements per ml, by performing a series of successive dilutions in their culture medium.

For each batch of cells thus obtained, four Corning containers were prepared in the following way:

- first two containers (control): 1 ml 20,000 elements/ml cell suspension, 1.4 ml of culture medium, 0.1 ml of sterile distilled water,

– other two containers (tests): 1 ml 20,000 elements/ml cell suspension, 1.4 ml of culture medium, 0.1 ml of mercury chloride solution n° 2.

After being homogenized, all containers were set in a stove to be sterilized at 37° C for 48 hours, and the mitotic index was determined as described in the "determination of the subtoxic dose" section.

The whole of these operations is shown on Chart III.

Chart III

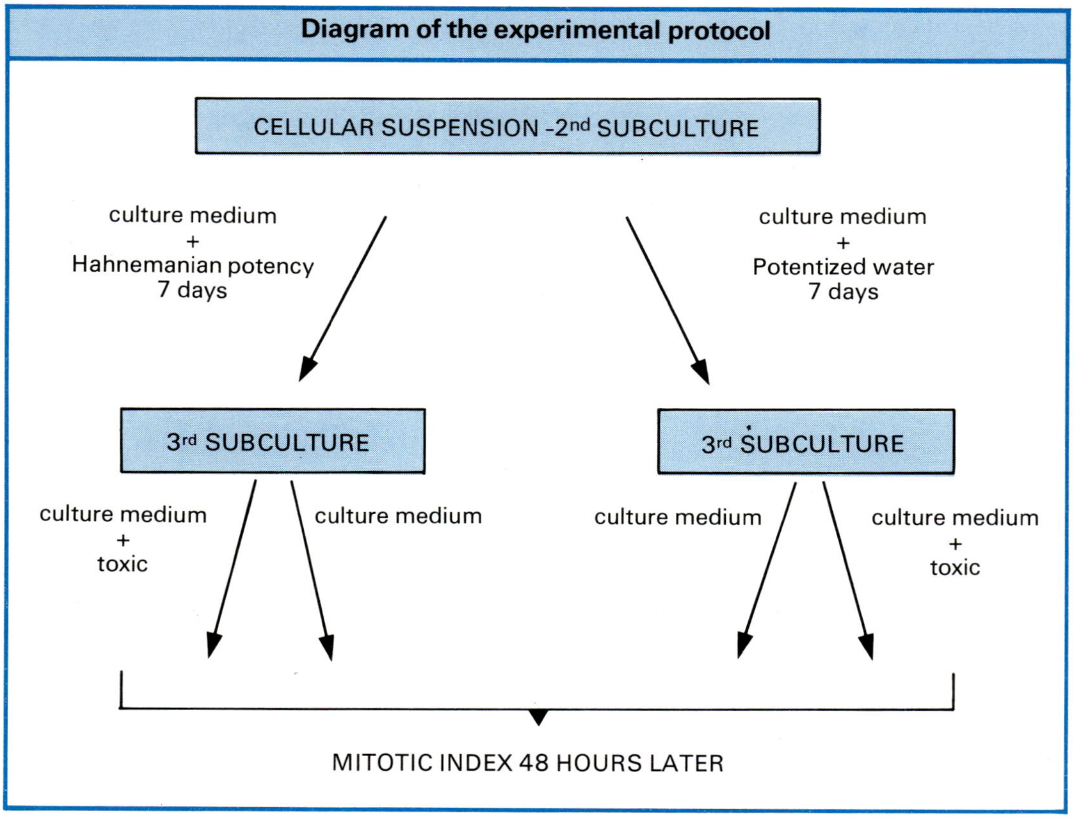

ANALYZED RESULTS

1. DETERMINATION OF THE SUB-TOXIC DOSE

Chart IV shows the whole of mitotic index figures for each of the Corning containers, whether they were treated or not treated with the mercury chloride solution at 1/160,000 and 1/180,000.

It shows that the addition of mercury chloride at 1/180,000 brings a lowering of the mitotic index to 47%. We consequently retained this concentration as being a sub-toxic dose.

Chart IV

Determination of the sub-toxic dose compared to mitotic index figures					
Strains	**Control**	**Trial 1 Mercurius corrosivus 1/160 000**	**Decrease of mitotic index**	**Trial 2 Mercurius corrosivus 1/180 000**	**Decrease of mitotic index**
1243 F 01	Ta 3.3 Tb 3.1 → 3.2	trial a : 1.4 trial b : 1.3	56 % 59 %	trial a : 1.5 trial b : 1.8	53 % 44 %
1244 F 01	Ta 2.9 Tb 3.1 → 3	trial a : 1.5 trial b : 1.6	50 % 47 %	trial a : 1.6 trial b : 1.8	47 % 40 %
1303 F 01	Ta 3.9 Tb 4.4 → 4.15	trial a : 1 trial b : 1.1	76 % 73.5 %	trial a : 1.96 trial b : 1.94	53 % 53 %
1304 F 01	Ta 3.2 Tb 3 → 3.1	trial a : 1.25 trial b : 1.4	60 % 55 %	trial a : 1.6 trial b : 1.55	48 % 50 %
1310 F 01	Ta 3.8 Tb 4 → 3.9	trial a : 1.25 trial b : damaged slide	68 %	trial a : 1.8 trial b : 2	54 % 49 %
1219 F 01	Ta 2.5 Tb 2.7 → 2.6	trial a : 1.1 trial b : 1.3	58 % 50 %	trial a : 1.9 trial b : 1.8	27 % 31 %
1343 F 01	Ta 2.2 Tb 2.1 → 2.15	trial a : 0.89 trial b : 0.88	59 % 59 %	trial a : 1.06 trial b : 1.16	51 % 46 %
Average	**3.157**	**1.228**	**61 %**	**1.676**	**47 %**

2. TESTS ON HAHNEMANIAN POTENCIES

Chart V includes mitotic index figures for each of the Corning containers previously treated either with 5 C Potentized Water or with 5 C Mercurius corrosivus, for one week.

It shows that, in the presence of 5 C Potentized Water, the mitotic index decreases by 41.37% on an average, whereas in the presence of 5 C Mercurius corrosivus, the mitotic index decreases by 34.79% on an average.

Chart VI includes mitotic index figures for each of the Corning containers previously treated either with 15 C Potentized Water or with 15 C Mercurius corrosivus for one week.

It shows that, in the presence of 15 C Potentized Water, the mitotic index decreases by 34.7% on an average, whereas in the presence of 15 C Mercurius corrosivus, the mitotic index decreases by 35.76% on an average.

Chart V

Strains	Cells treated with 5 C Potentized water for one week			Cells treated with 5 C Mercurius corrosivus for one week		
	Control	Hg Cl_2 trial 1/180,000	Decrease of mitotic index	Control	Hg Cl_2 trial 1/180,000	Decrease of mitotic index
1343 F 01 Sub. 2	2.28 2.40 → 2.34	1.06	55 %	2.47 2.60 → 2.53	1.08 1.06 → 1.07	58 %
1347 F 01 Sub. 2	2.80 2.80 → 2.80	1.76 1.80 → 1.78	36.5 %	2.80 3.30 → 3.05	2.20 2.48 → 2.34	23 %
1379 F 01 Sub. 2	2.78 2.75 → 2.76	1.44 1.40 → 1.42	49 %	3.00 2.80 → 2.90	2.00 1.65 → 1.82	37 %
1415 F 01 Sub. 2	1.96 2.00 → 1.98	1.33 1.30 → 1.31	34 %	2.00 2.00 → 2.00	1.65 1.56 → 1.60	20 %
1414 F 01 Sub. 2	3.00 2.50 → 2.75	2.00 1.74 → 1.87	32 %	2.95	1.33 1.50 → 1.41	52.20 %
1432 F 01 Sub. 2	2.00 2.00 → 2.00	1.05 1.00 → 1.02	49 %	1.80 1.90 → 1.85	1.20 1.00 → 1.10	40.50 %
1403 F 01 Sub. 2	1.77 1.89 → 1.83	1.16 1.07 → 1.11	40 %	1.76 1.80 → 1.78	1.10 1.14 → 1.12	38 %
1467 F 01 Sub. 2	2.26 2.08 → 2.17	1.42 1.40 → 1.41	35 %	2.45 2.15 → 2.30	1.64 1.45 → 1.55	33 %
1481 F 01 Sub. 2	1.90 2.00 → 1.95	1.20 1.00 → 1.10	44 %	1.96 1.82 → 1.89	1.50 1.53 → 1.51	21 %
1482 F 01 Sub. 2	2.06 1.76 → 1.81	0.90 0.86 → 0.88	54 %	2.20 1.16 → 2.18	1.45 1.48 → 1.46	33 %
1525 F 01 Sub. 2	2.04 2.32 → 2.18	1.67 1.48 → 1.57	28 %	2.40 2.00 → 2.20	1.65 1.63 → 1.64	26 %
1495 F 01 Sub. 2	2.56 2.60 → 2.58	1.55 1.56 → 1.55	40 %	2.76 3.00 → 2.78	1.90 1.65 → 1.77	36 %
Average	**2.27**	**1.35**	**41.37 %**	**2.30**	**1.53**	**34.79 %**

Table title: **Level of mitotic index for cultures treated with either 5 C Potentized water or with 5 C Mercurius corrosivus**

Chart VI

Level of mitotic index for cultures treated with either 15 C Potentized water or with 15 C Mercurius corrosivus						
Strains	**Cells treated with 15 C Potentized water for one week**			**Cells treated with 15 C Mercurius corrosivus for one week**		
	Control	**Hg Cl_2 trial 1/180,000**	**Decrease of mitotic index**	**Control**	**Hg Cl_2 trial 1/180,000**	**Decrease of mitotic index**
1343 F 01 Sub. 2	2.11 2.22 → 2.16	0.91 1.00 → 0.95	56 %	2.40 2.21 → 2.30	1.00 1.09 → 1.04	55.60 %
1347 F 01 Sub. 2	2.25 2.25 → 2.25	1.70 1.55 → 1.62	28 %	2.40 2.30 → 2.35	1.95 1.85 → 1.90	20 %
1379 F 01 Sub. 2	2.38 2.30 → 2.34	1.60 1.50 → 1.55	34 %	2.40 2.60 → 2.50	1.73 1.62 → 1.67	33 %
1415 F 01 Sub. 2	2.50 2.80 → 2.65	1.72 1.77 → 1.74	34 %	2.50 2.50 → 2.50	1.69 1.50 → 1.59	36 %
1414 F 01 Sub. 2	4.00 4.20 → 4.10	2.20 2.00 → 2.10	49 %	4.00 4.20 → 4.10	1.80 2.00 → 1.90	54 %
1467 F 01 Sub. 2	2.31 2.35 → 2.33	1.58 1.70 → 1.64	30 %	2.30 2.34 → 2.32	1.50 1.32 → 1.41	39 %
1481 F 01 Sub. 2	1.72 1.68 → 1.70	1.40 1.36 → 1.38	19 %	1.76 1.73 → 1.74	1.34 1.47 → 1.40	20 %
1482 F 01 Sub. 2	1.91 2.00 → 1.95	1.00 1.10 → 1.05	47 %	2.10 1.80 → 1.95	0.88 1.00 → 0.94	52 %
1525 F 01 Sub. 2	2.10 2.33 → 2.21	1.76 1.73 → 1.74	21 %	2.18 2.29 → 2.23	1.72 1.87 → 1.79	20 %
1495 F 01 Sub. 2	2.46 2.50 → 2.48	1.75 1.78 → 1.76	29 %	2.21 2.33 → 2.27	1.59 1.69 → 1.64	28 %
Average	**2.42**	**1.55**	**34.50 %**	**2.43**	**1.53**	**35.40 %**

DISCUSSION

For each of the Hahnemanian potencies tested, four results were obtained:

- a mitotic index corresponding to cells treated with Potentized Water only (index 1);
- a mitotic index corresponding to cells treated with Potentized Water containing a sub-toxic dose of mercury chloride (index 2);
- a mitotic index corresponding to cells treated with Hahnemanian potencies only (index 3);
- a mitotic index corresponding to cells treated with a Hahnemanian potency, then having received a sub-toxic dose of mercury chloride (index 4).

1. THE CASE OF 5 C MERCURIUS CORROSIVUS

Upon reading the results obtained during these tests, it appeared that figures of mitotic indexes 1 and 3 were almost identical, and that the only figures to vary were those of mitotic indexes 2 and 4.

Applying of the Wilcoxon T test made it possible to evaluate the significant character of the results. For each cell strain, we calculated the difference between mitotic indexes 2 and 4 by attributing a plus (+) sign to the figure when the difference was in favor of mitotic index n° 4, and a minus sign (–) in the opposite case.

Results thus obtained were classified by order of absolute increasing value as shown in Chart VII. By referring to Wilcoxon's table, it appeared that, for 12 trials, the lower limit for T (sum total of the ranks of differences in minus signs) at a threshold of 5% was 14.

Chart VII

Results obtained with 5 C Mercurius corrosivus, expressed using Wilcoxon's table

Strains	Differences between mitotic index 2 and 4	Rank
1343 F 01	+ 0.01	2
1347 F 01	+ 0.56	12
1379 F 01	+ 0.40	8
1415 F 01	+ 0.29	7
1414 F 01	– 0.46	10
1432 F 01	+ 0.08	4
1403 F 01	+ 0.01	1
1467 F 01	+ 0.14	5
1481 F 01	+ 0.41	9
1482 F 01	+ 0.58	11
1525 F 01	+ 0.07	3
1495 F 01	+ 0.22	6

And yet, in this precise case, the only minus sign figure to be found has a rank of 10, thus making it possible to state that our figures were significant at a threshold of 5%; we can consequently assert with a degree of probability higher than 95% that the preventive treatment with Mercurius corrosivus 5 C favorably influences the in culture multiplication of fibroblasts intoxicated with mercury chloride.

2. THE CASE OF 15 C. MERCURIUS CORROSIVUS

By applying Wilcoxon's T test to the figures of mitotic indexes 2 and 4, we obtained Chart VIII. According to Wilcoxon's table, the lower limit of T at the threshold of 5% was 8 for 10 trials. And yet in this case, T being valued at 33, the results would not be considered as significant, and the treatment with 15 C Mercurius corrosivus could not, as a consequence, be considered as effective.

Chart VIII

Results obtained with 15 C Mercurius corrosivus, expressed in accordance with wilcoxon

Strains	Difference between mitotic indexes 2 and 4	Rank
1343 F 01	+ 0.09	3
1347 F 01	+ 0.28	10
1379 F 01	+ 0.12	6
1415 F 01	− 0.15	7
1414 F 01	− 0.20	8
1467 F 01	− 0.23	9
1481 F 01	+ 0.02	1
1482 F 01	− 0.11	4
1525 F 01	+ 0.05	2
1495 F 01	− 0.12	5

We felt that this text was interesting to study in that it corroborated, on the cellular level, a whole series of coordinated facts, now well-established "in vivo" in plants and whole animals, namely that a Hahnemanian potency of a toxic substance had a protective effect against this same toxic substance.

It is to be noted that these toxic concentrations and concentrations having a protective effect against this toxic action are in relation of 10^7, respectively, 2.10^{-5} M and 6.5 10^{-12} M.

This type of study is currently carried out in order to investigate the effects of other Mercurius corrosivus potencies.

SECTION V

THE EFFECTS OF 7 C HISTAMINUM AND 7 C APIS MELLIFICA HAHNEMANIAN POTENCIES UPON BASOPHIL DEGRANULATION IN ALLERGIC PATIENTS

INTRODUCTION

Among the biological processes evidenced and analyzed in the course of the past 50 years, the allergic reaction is one of those which would seem to have the greatest number of clinical applications, while retaining a fundamental interest at the same time. To prove this, we need only consider the proliferation of allergology societies and the growing number of publications and congresses devoted to this speciality.

For homeopaths, the interest taken in following the results and developments of this biological and therapeutical method is greater than for the average practitioner, as they are more able to cast an attentive and critical judgement upon a technique which is in many ways close to their own as regards doses used and concepts involved.

We first of all decided to eliminate the individual character of the patient's reaction to the remedy, as it is contrary to a statistical interpretation of the results and might have induced serious criticism of the method. We selected a perfectly quantifiable, biological method realized in vitro likely to be used for the development of the same kind of studies in human clinical medicine, should the results prove positive.

The degranulation test with human TDBH basophils seemed to meet the expressed requirements.

If the basophils having anaphylactic antibodies fixed to their membranal receptors are in contact with antigens at a temperature of 37° C, they degranulate, in other words, they liberate the contents of their cytoplasmic granules into the extra-cellular medium: pre-formed or neo-formed mediators.

This type of reaction is evidenced when immediate hypersensivity (type 1) according to the Gell and Combs classification, appears. The basophils which have degranulated are distinguishable from those not having degranulated by the loss of their metachromatic tinctorial affinity with Toluidine blue.

This test, defined by J. Benveniste consists of setting the patient's basophils, obtained by performing a concentration of a blood sample, in contact with the suspected allergen, the latter being first dried on a microtitration plate. Six potencies of this allergen, from 10 to 10, were systematically compared to two controls containing no allergen.

Basophils, which are stainable in Toluidine blue before they are put in contact with the allergen are no longer so after liberating the mediators. The use of six potencies of the allergen makes it possible to find the optimum concentration zone in every case, and also to avoid zone phenomena.

A statistical calculation based on the application of Poisson's law, makes it possible to define a significance threshold which, on an average, is situated between 20 and 35%, depending on the number of basophils counted.

The trial consisted of performing a series of basophil degranulation tests. Each of these tests was conducted once in, and once out of the presence of the Hahnemanian potency the effect of which upon TDBH was to be confirmed.

The studied potencies were selected in order to stay as close as possible to the Law of Similars. Knowing that histamine is one of the main constituents of the basophils' granules, we studied the effect of 7 C Histaminum.

Besides, we studied the effect of 7 C Apis Mellifica in patients allergic to hymenopters.

The controls were, in every case, sterile distilled water in a corresponding potency.

MATERIAL AND METHODS

1. THE BASOPHILS' DEGRANULATION TEST TECHNIQUE

The Hahnemanian potency to be studied was introduced at 9/10 in a buffer called the basophils' buffer washer solution. The complement to 10 was a mineral buffer solution (medium A).

The basophils contained in the sample were centrifuged at a very low speed, resuspended in medium A and pre-incubated for 20 mn at 37° C in a medium containing the ions needed for causing the degranulation reaction (Ca^{++} and Mg^{++}), and the human serum albumin.

An aliquot of this concentration was then used in order to perform the TDBH.

In order to perform this, 10 microlitres of the basophil suspension were placed inside the cupules of a microtitration plate in the lower part of which the antigen was previously dried. After 15 mn of incubation at 37° C, the basophils not having degranulated were counted by putting them in contact with an acid solution of Toluidine blue.

Six potencies of the antigen were systematically tested. A bell shaped curve with its two inhibition zones due to excess antibodies and antigens was thus generally obtained.

The maximum percentage of degranulation was then calculated.

2. THE HAHNEMANIAN POTENCIES

They were prepared in sterile distilled water, in order to avoid possible interferences with traces of alcohol in the basophils' degranulation test.

Sixty-seven degranulation tests were performed in patients whose results were positive regarding various allergens in the case of Histaminum, and wasp and bee venom in the case of Apis mellifica.

The allergens selected for the Histaminum trials were both proteins (mold, mites, dermoskeleton, retinal antigens) and drugs. Certain of these allergens were haptenes.

ANALYZED RESULTS

The result was expressed in % of degranulation, the threshold of statistical significance being determined according to the number of cells counted.

Results are to be found in Charts I, II, III, IV. Both figures in column 2 and 4 represent the number of cells compared for the control, and the optimum allergen concentration, respectively with and without the studied product.

Whenever the percentage of degranulation is lower than the level of significance, this is indicated as "NS", e.g. non significant.

Every time basophils' degranulation was inhibited, the trial also became un-significant (US).

1. TRIALS CARRIED OUT WITH 7 C HISTAMINUM

These trials demonstrated that this Hahnemanian potency completely blocked the in vitro human basophils's degranulation in a large majority of cases (76%).

In half the remaining cases, that is 12% of the studied cases, the blocking was well-defined, however incomplete.

Under the experimental conditions used here, 7 C Histaminum thus remained with no effect in 12% of the studied cases only.

Chart I

7 C Histaminum						
Allergens	Count of basophils without Hist.		% of degranulation	Count of basophils without Hist.		% of degranulation
Aspirin	33	17	50	16	12	NS
Paracetamol	35	25	31	54	50	NS
Bilharziasis	30	7	80	31	26	NS
Shrimp	26	13	50	31	29	NS
Orgametril	43	25	42	40	27	32
Telebrix	41	25	39	39	23	41
Aspirin	49	25	51	44	46	NS
Cat hair	21	8	62	20	18	NS
Aspergillus	33	3	90	41	30	27
Retinal antigens	33	16	51	28	28	NS
Mold	38	20	47	28	21	NS
Pollen	25	6	76	17	16	NS
Anesthetics	29	8	72	20	11	45
Anesthetics	25	9	56	15	15	NS
Mosquito	26	14	46	26	24	NS
Candida albicans	25	9	56	15	15	NS
Household dust	28	8	68	14	14	NS
Aspirin	60	35	42	30	29	NS
Mold	38	17	55	16	16	25
Mites	56	27	53	24	23	NS
Acarians	41	16	61	32	29	NS
Penicillin G	56	27	52	18	10	44
Streptococcus	49	34	30	32	30	NS
Insects	28	12	57	12	5	58
Mites	71	43	39	40	40	NS
Tartrazine	38	17	55	16	17	NS
E 122	29	11	62	20	16	NS
Erythrosine	39	14	64	19	17	NS
Candida albicans	74	45	40	25	26	NS
Aspirin	66	45	32	27	27	NS
Ampicillin	49	26	47	27	24	NS
Xylocaine	43	22	49	29	28	NS
Scandicaine	28	13	53	43	28	35
Mites	47	17	64	25	24	NS

2. TRIALS CARRIED OUT WITH 7 C APIS MELLIFICA

As regards these trials, the number of cases studied was smaller, this being owed to a mere recruitment problem. However, conclusions comparable to the ones drawn from the former trial could appear.

Chart II

7 C Apis mellifica						
Allergens	**Count of basophils without Apis**		**% of degranulation**	**Count of basophils with Apis**		**% of degranulation**
Wasp	18	6	67	17	11	35
Bee	22	10	54	13	13	NS
Wasp	29	5	83	34	35	NS
Bee	23	11	52	41	38	NS
Wasp	35	6	83	38	16	58
Wasp	33	13	61	18	18	NS
Bee	50	20	60	15	6	60

3. OTHER TRIALS CARRIED OUT WITH 7 C HISTAMINUM

Other trials were undertaken with 7 C Histaminum, in double blind, with different manufacturing batches.

Batches 1257, 21888 and 1294 were verum. Batch 1293 was a distilled water placebo. These results clearly confirmed those shown on Chart I.

On an average, for batches 1257 and 21888, 75% of the degranulation were completely blocked by 7 C Histaminum, in other words, the percentage of degranulation obtained after incubation with 7 C Histaminum became un-statistically significant. It is to be noted that this activity was observed for haptenes, as well as for multivalent antigens.

In the course of the comparative trial carried out on different batches of 7 C Histaminum, one of the two batches was found to have a stronger activity than the other (Chart III). The difference was not, however, significant.

In the trial carried out on two ordinary batches (Chart IV) one of which was distilled water, the blockage was systematically observed with the same batch (7 C Histaminum) whereas the other (7 C distilled Water) showed no activity whatsoever.

Chart III

Comparative trials of two batches of 7 C Histaminum expressed in % of degranulation			
Allergens	**Without 7 C Histaminum**	**Batch 1257**	**Batch 21888**
Cow's milk	33	NS	NS
Aspirin	62	NS	NS
Retina	67	NS	50
Unidone	35	NS	NS
Procaine	44	NS	24
Tromexane	44	NS	56

Chart IV

Comparative trials of two ordinary batches expressed in % of degranulation 1293 : 7 C distilled water - 1294 : Histaminum 7 C			
Allergens	**Without Hahnem. potency**	**Batch 1293**	**Batch 1294**
Zyloric	45	56	NS
Nickel	80	88	NS
Cochineal red	50	56	NS
Cefalotine	58	50	NS
Rimifon	72	55	NS
Tetracycline	52	56	NS
Madecassol	60	46	NS
Geotrichum	55	37	44

DISCUSSION

With 7 C Histaminum, we obtained 76% of totally positive results 12% of partially positive results, and only 12% of negative results.

This is all the more remarkable that substances which are currently on the market do not allow to obtain results corresponding to more than 25% of positive cases in the basophils degranulation test.

With 7 C Apis mellifica, given the more restricted number of blood samples, it was obviously more difficult to come to a conclusion, in spite of the fact that the anti-degranulating activity was very clear.

7 C Histaminum and 7 C Apis mellifica, do therefore, have an anti-degranulating activity "in vitro", with reference to the experimental model used by us.

Can it be attributed to a negative feed-back from histamine on the level of the corresponding membranal receptors, the existence of which has clearly been proved?

BIBLIOGRAPHY

BALDESSARINI R.J., KAROBATH H. – Biochemical physiology of central synapses - Ann. Rev. Physiol. 35 (1973) 273-304.

BIRD E.D., SPOKES E.G., IVERSEN L.L. – Increased Dopamine Concentration in limbic areas of Brain from patients Dying with Schizophrenia. Brain 102 (1979) 347-360.

BOIRON J., CIER A. – Elimination provoquée et spécificité d'action des dilutions infinitésimales d'éléments toxiques.
Annales homéopathiques françaises (1962) 10, 789-795.

BRUINVELS J. – Role of sodium in neuronal uptake of monoamines and aminoacid precursor Nature 257 (1975) 606-607.

CIER A., BOIRON J., VINGER Ch., BRAISE J. – Sur le traitement du diabète expérimental par des dilutions infinitésimales d'alloxane.
Annales homéopathiques françaises (1966) 2, 137-145.

COOPER J.R., BLOOM F.E., ROTH R.H. – The biochemical basis of Neuropharmacology. Oxford University Press (1978).

CUEILLERON P., FONLUPT P., PACHECO H. – Effets de la teinture de Gelsemium sur la capture de la dopamine, de la noradrénaline et de la sérotonine dans des préparations synaptosomales du cerveau de rat (CR. Acad. Sc. Paris, t. 294 - 19 avril 1982).

GORNALL A.G., BARDAWILL C.J., DAVID M.M. – Determination of serum proteins by means of the biuret reaction. J. Biol. Chem. 177 (1949) 751-766.

HALL Z.W., HILDEBRAND J.C., KRAVITZ E.A. – The Chemistry of synaptic Transmission essays and sources. Chinon Press (1974).

HENN F.A., HAMBERGER A. – Glial cell function : Uptake of transmitter substances. Proc. Nat. Acad. Sci. 68 (1971) 2686-2690.

IVERSEN L.L. – Dopamine Receptors in the Brain : A dopamine-sensitive adenylatecyclate models synaptic receptors, illuminating antipsychotic drug action. Science 188 (1975) 1084-1089.

IVERSEN S.D., IVERSEN L.L. – Behavioral Pharmacology. Oxford University Press 2nd ed. (1980).

JOUANNY J. – Notions essentielles de Matière Médicale Homéopathique. Les Laboratoires Boiron Editeur 5e Ed. Lyon (1979).

LABORIT H., HUGUENARD P., ALLUAUME R. – Un nouveau stabilisateur végétatif (LE 4560 RP) Presse Médicale 60 (1952) 206-208.

LAPP C., WURMSER L., NEY J. – Mobilisation de l'arsenic fixe chez le cobaye sous l'influence de doses infinitésimales d'arseniate de sodium. Thérapie (1955) 10 - 625-638.

MOURIQUAND G., CIER A., BOIRON J., EDEL V., CHIGHIZOLA R. – Variations de l'indice chronologique vestibulaire et de l'élimination arsenicale chez le pigeon sous l'effet de doses infinitésimales d'arsenic. Assises pour la recherche scientifique en homéopathie. Lyon 18 mars 1961 - 19-34.

NETIEN G., BOIRON J., MARIN A. – Action de doses infinitésimales de sulfate de cuivre sur des plantes préalablement intoxiquées par cette substance.
Annales homéopathiques françaises (1966) - 2 - 130.

NIOULHON A., CHERAMY A., GLOWINSKI. – An adaptation of the Push-pull cannula method to study the in vivo release of H3 Dopamine synthesized from H3 Tyrosine in the cat caudate nucleus : effect of various physical and pharmacological treatements. J. Neurochem 28 (1977) 819-828.

SCHWARTZ M.B., PIRO L., LAJTHA A. – Relationship of ATP levels to aminoacid transport in slice of mouse brain. Arch. Biochem. Biophys. 145 (1971) 199-210.

SHASKAN E.G., SNYDER S.H. – Kinetics of serotonin accumulation into slices from rat brain : relationship to catecholamine uptake. J. Pharm. - Exp. Therap. 175 (1970) 404.418.

SNYDER S.H., COYLE J.T. – Regional differences in H3 norepinephrine and H3 dopamine uptake into rat brain homogenates. J. Pharm. Exp. Therap. 165 (1969) 78-86.

SUPPLEMENT

International bibliography
in the Field of homeopathy

Trials carried out in France

ABREVIATIONS

A.H.F. : Annales Homéopathiques Françaises.

H.G. : The Hahnemannian Gleanings.

B.H.J. : The British Homeopathic Journal.

J.A.I.H. : Journal of the American Institute of Homeopathy.

R.B.H. : Revue Belge d'Homeopathie.

A.H.Z. : Allgemeine Homöopathische Zeitung.

C.H.F. : Centre Homéopathique de France.

C.H.T.C. : Cahiers d'Homéopathie et de Thérapie comparée.

L.H.M.I. : Ligue Médicale Homéopathique Internationale.

ANTHONY J. – Considérations sur la systématique des serpents à l'usage des médecins homéopathes.
A.H.F., 1962.

AUBIN M. – Objectivation expérimentale de l'action d'un médicament homéopathique.
Communication faite aux XIIe Assises scientifiques homéopathiques du Touquet, 1973.

AUBIN M. – Toxicologie et expérimentation animale : étude de l'action hépatotoxique du Phosphore blanc.
Communication faite au Congrès des Sociétés médicales homéopathiques, Paris, octobre 1975.

AUBIN M., BARONNET S., CHAZAUD J., BURANTIN G., VILLIE F. et BASTIDE P. – Action de diverses dilutions d'Arnica sur les taux de lactate déshydrogénase et de malate déshydrogénase du muscle de rats soumis à une épreuve d'effort.
Communication faite aux XVe Assises scientifiques homéopathiques, à Dijon, 30 avril 1976.

AUBIN M., BARONNET S., BASTIDE P. et BASTIDE J. – Etude pharmacologique d'une préparation d'Apis 7 CH vis-à-vis de l'érythème aux rayons ultra-violets chez le cobaye albinos. (Travail du service de Pharmacologie et de Biochimie de la Faculté de médecine et de pharmacie de Clermont-Ferrand).
A.H.F. Communication faite aux XIVe Assises scientifiques homéopathiques, mai 1975.

AUBIN M. et BILDET J. – Homéopathie et expérimentation animale : Méthode générale (Aubin) - Etude de l'action de différentes dilutions homéopathiques de Phosphore blanc (Phosphorus) sur l'hépatite toxique du rat (Thèse Bildet).
La Documentation homéopathique, 1975.

BAGROS M. – Phénomènes d'antagonismes et de synergie entre diverses dilutions de folliculine.
Actes de la Société Rhodanienne d'Homéopathie, juillet 1952.

BARANGER et FILER M.-K. – Essai de traitement de la leucémie aviaire (lymphomatose) par les dilutions homéopathiques de méthycholanthrène, de pseudo-cantharidine et d'isosulfocyanate d'allyle.
A.H.F. n° 8, 1965.

BARANGER et FILER K. – Contribution à l'étude de différents facteurs pouvant influer sur l'efficacité des dilutions homéopathiques.
A.H.F., 1967.

BARANGER et FILER K. – Contribution à l'étude des facteurs pouvant influer sur l'efficacité thérapeutique des dilutions homéopathiques.
A.H.F., 1968.

BARANGER et FILER M.-K. – Comparaison des activités thérapeutiques des mêmes substances à doses allopathiques et homéopathiques.
A.H.F., 1968.

BARBIER M. – Pour une pharmacologie homéopathique.
Bulletin du Syndicat national des médecins homéopathes français, 1969 juillet-août.

BEJA A. – L'action biologique des dilutions infinitésimales homéopathiques de corps œstrogènes et ses conséquences thérapeutiques.
Thèse médecine, Paris juin 1953.

BILDET J., BONINI F., GENDRE Ph., AUBIN M., DEMARQUE D. et QUILICHINI R. – Etude au microscope électronique de l'action de dilutions de Phosphorus 15 CH sur l'hépatite toxique du rat.
Communication faite aux XVe Assises scientifiques homéopathiques à Dijon, avril 1976.

BILDET J., GUERE J.M., SAUREL J., AUBIN M., DEMARQUE D. et QUILICHINI R. – Etude de l'action préventive de différentes dilutions de Phosphorus sur l'hépatite toxique du rat. (Travail du Laboratoire de Pharmacologie de la Faculté de Médecine et de Pharmacie de Bordeaux).
Communication faite aux XIVe Assises scientifiques homéopathiques de mai 1975.

BILDET J., GUERE J.M., SAUREL J., AUBIN M., DEMARQUE D. et QUILICHINI R. – Etude de l'action curative de différentes dilutions de Phosphorus sur l'hépatite toxique du rat. (Travail du Laboratoire de Pharmacologie de la Faculté de Médecine et de Pharmacie de Bordeaux).
Communication faite aux XIVe Assises scientifiques homéopathiques de mai 1975.

BOFFA M.C. – Vipera Apis - Effets cliniques et biologiques du venin chez l'homme.
A.H.F. n° 5, 1970.

BOFFA M.C. – Modification du complément sérique par le venin de Naja Nigricollis (absorption per linguale de dose infinitésimale).
A.H.F. n° 2, 1976.

BOFFA M.C. – Expérimentation du venin de Naja Nigricollis.
A.H.F. n° 5, 1976.

BOIRON H. et BAGROS M. – Etude de dilutions de folliculine à la 30ᵉ CH.
Actes Congrès de la Société Rhodanienne, 1955.

BOIRON H., BAGROS M. et DANEL. – Etude expérimentale de l'activité biologique de dilutions homéopathiques croissantes de Folliculine.
Actes de la Société Rhodanienne d'Homéopathie, 1955.

BOIRON J. – Contrôle de l'imprégnation des granules homéopathiques à l'aide de produits marqués.
A.H.F. 1961.

BOIRON J. – Action de dilutions homéopathiques de $HgCl_2$ sur la respiration des coléoptiles de blé.
A.H.F. n° 4, 1965.

BOIRON J. – Action d'une dilution hahnemannienne arsenicale sur la croissance du blé intoxiqué à l'arsenic.
A.H.F. n° 4, 1965.

BOIRON J. – Effets diabétogènes de l'Alloxane 7 CH, 9 CH, 15 CH et 30 CH sur le diabète alloxanique provoqué.
Congrès de la L.H.M.I. Vienne, 1973.

BOIRON J. et BRAISE J. – Nouvelle technique de préparation des dilutions korsakoviennes. Etude de la déconcentration des dilutions à l'aide d'un produit marqué.
A.H.F., 1965.

BOIRON J. et CIER A. – Recherches expérimentales d'une activité isopathique.
A.H.F., 1962.

BOIRON J. et CIER A. – Etudes de quelques propriétés biologiques du sérum d'anguille.
A.H.F., 1962.

BOIRON J. et CIER A. – Influence de différents facteurs physiques sur l'activité pharmacodynamique des dilutions infinitésimales.
IXᵉ Assises scientifiques homéopathiques, mai 1970.

BOIRON J., CIER A. et NETIEN G. – Dix ans de recherches en Homéopathie.
A.H.F. n° 11, 1971.

BOIRON J., CIER A., VINGERT C. – Effets de quelques facteurs physiques sur l'activité pharmacologique de dilutions infinitésimales.
A.H.F., 1968.

BOIRON J. et CUCHET. – Etude de quelques modifications dans la préparation des T.M. figurant à la pharmacopée.
A.H.F., 1967.

BOIRON J. et CUCHET. – Etude de quelques teintures-mères animales.
A.H.F., 1968.

BOIRON J. et MAILLOT D. – Premières recherches sur l'inactivité des dilutions préparées sous azote.
Xᵉ Assises scient. homéo. Strasbourg, 10 juin 1971.

BOIRON J. et MAILLOT D. – Etude pharmacodynamique d'un remède de l'asthénie et de la fatigue musculaire « sarcolactate de zinc ».
XIᵉ Assises scient. homéo. Bordeaux 20 avril 1972.

BOIRON J. et MARIN. – Action de deux dilutions successives de $HgCl_2$ sur la respiration des coléoptiles de blé.
A.H.F. n° 8, 1965.

BOIRON J., MARIN. – Actions de dilutions homéopathiques de Fluorure de Sodium sur la vitesse de réaction de l'Invertase.
A.H.F., 1965.

BOIRON J. et MARIN. – Action des doses infinitésimales (15 CH) d'une substance sur la cinétique d'élimination de cette même substance au cours de la culture de graines préalablement intoxiquées.
A.H.F. n° 2, 1967.

BOIRON J. et MARIN. – Action d'une 15 CH de SO CU sur la cinétique d'élimination de cette substance au cours de la culture « d'embryons » préalablement intoxiqués.
A.H.F., 1968.

BOIRON J. et MARIN. – Action d'une 15ᵉ CH de sulfate de cuivre sur la culture de chlorella vulgaris.
IXᵉ Assises scient. homéo. Vichy, 29 mai 1970.

BOIRON J. et VOLLE. – Contribution à l'étude du vieillissement des teintures-mères.
A.H.F., 1963.

BOIRON J. et ZERVUDACHI. – Action de dilutions infinitésimales d'arseniate de sodium sur la respiration de coléoptiles de blé.
A.H.F., 1963.

BONNET MAURY P., DAYSINE A. et VOEGELI M.L. – Etude des dilutions korsakoviennes par les radioisotopes.
A.H.F., 1954.

BROLLY S. – Etudes de dilutions de Gelsemium Sempervirens et de granules imprégnés de dilution de Gelsemium Sempervirens.
A.H.F., 1962.

CIER A. – Possibilités de recherche en Homéopathie.
Actualités homéopathiques.

CIER A., BOIRON J. – Elimination provoquée et spécificité d'action des dilutions infinitésimales d'éléments toxiques.
A.H.F., 1962.

CIER A., BOIRON J. – Pharmacologie homéopathique. Les possibilités de recherches sur les animaux préalablement sensibilisés.
A.H.F., 1967.

CIER A., BOIRON J. et QUENOT J. – Hépatites expérimentales et essais de médications homéopathiques.
A.H.F., 1963.

CIER A., BOIRON J. et QUENOT J. – Diabète alloxanique et dilutions infinitésimales d'alloxane.
A.H.F., 1965.

CIER A., BOIRON J. et VINGERT C. – Essais pharmacologiques de nouvelles dilutions korsakoviennes.
A.H.F., 1965.

CIER A., BOIRON J., VINGERT C. et BRAISE J. – Sur le traitement du diabète expérimental par des dilutions infinitésimales d'alloxane.
A.H.F., 1966.

CIER A., GIRARD, ROUSSON Ch. et BOIRON J. – Intoxication arsenicale et élimination provoquée d'arsenic.
A.H.F., 1963-1964.

COLAS H., AUBIN M., PICARD Ph. et BASTIDE J. – Inhibition du test de transformation lymphoblasti-

que par Phytolacca en dilution homéopathique. (Travail effectué dans le laboratoire de virologie immunologique de la Faculté de médecine et de pharmacie de Montpellier).
Communication faite aux XIVe Assises scientifiques homéopathiques, mai 1975.

DANO. – Action désensibilisante de hautes dilutions d'un dérivé diméthylé de la para-phénylène diamine.
A.H.F., 1963.

DAUDEL et ROBILLARD. – Etude des dilutions hahnemanniennes par la méthode des radio-isotopes.
Acad. de Pharm. séance du 2 juin 1954.

DEVRAIGNE, BAGROS, BOIRON et DESPAX. – Note sur un antagonisme pharmacodynamique entre des doses fortes et faibles d'une même substance hormonale.
Revue Franç. d'Homéopathie n° 3, 1953.

DEVRAIGNE, BAGROS et BOIRON H. – Etude expérimentale de l'activité biologique de dilutions homéopathiques de folliculine.
Communication faite à la Société rhodanienne d'Homéopathie en 1955.

DUCASSOU et POURET et Mme TEULE et CAZENAVE. – Expérimentations en cours sur l'appareil à dynamisations korsakoviennes.
XIe Assises scient. Homéo. Bordeaux 20 avril, 1972.

GIRARDET E. – Etude de dilutions de Chelidonium majus et de granules imprégnés de dilutions de Chelidonium majus.
A.H.F., 1962.

GRAVIOU. – Action d'une 15e centésimale de $CuSO_4$ sur la respiration de pois intoxiqués au cuivre.
A.H.F. n° 4, 1970.

GRAVIOU, BIRON A. – Action d'une 15e CH de sulfate de cuivre sur Lepidium en germination.
IXe Assises scient. Homéo. Vichy 29 mai 1970.

GRAVIOU, MARIN et collaborateurs. – Action de doses infinitésimales de sulfate de cuivre sur des plantes préalablement intoxiquées par cette substance.
A.H.F. n° 4, 1965.

HEINTZ E. – Nouvelles expériences sur le mode d'action de dilutions successives.
IXe Assises scient. Homéo. Vichy, 29 mai 1970.

HEINTZ E. – La mesure de l'action de dilutions successives à l'aide de piles électriques.
Xe Assises scient. Homéo. Homéo. Strasbourg, 10 juin 1971.

HEINTZ E. – Vérification expérimentale de la Loi d'Arndt Schultz.
Nouvelles expériences sur le mode d'action de dilutions successives.

HINSDALE. – Preuve scientifique de la valeur de la thérapeutique homéopathique illustrée par l'action de Mercurius cyanatus et de la toxine diphtérique.
A.H.F., 1950.

HUI BON HOA J. – Cantharis - Essai d'explication de son mécanisme d'action à doses infinitésimales.
A.H.F., mars 1968.

JARRICOT J. – Recherches expérimentales de test pour estimer l'activité du remède homéopathique.
Le Propagateur, 1932.

JARRICOT J. – Essais de critériums physiologiques pour mesurer l'activité du remède homéopathique.
Le Propagateur, 1933.

JARRICOT J. – Le travail musculaire commandé électriquement, comme test de l'activité de dynamisations homéopathiques et comme terme de comparaison de dilutions entre elles.
A.H.F., 1937.

JARRICOT J. – Aspect diphasique de toute action pharmacodynamique.
Actes de la Société Rhodanienne d'Homéopathie, septembre 1949.

JARRICOT J. – Iberis amara (expérimentation pharmacologique).
Actes de la Société Rhodanienne d'Homéopathie, mai 1951.

JARRICOT J. – Mécanisme de l'action du semblable.
Actes de la Société Rhodanienne d'Homéopathie n° 1, 1957.

JARRICOT J. – Trente ans d'études expérimentales appliquées à l'Homéopathie.
A.H.F., 1961.

JARRICOT J. – Les dilutions successives d'une substance soluble n'épuisent pas l'action spécifique de la substance, fut-elle déconcentrée bien au-delà du seuil où théoriquement les dernières molécules devraient avoir disparu.
A.H.F., 1962.

JEANNES, TETAU et FOUCHE. – Expérimentation pharmacologique de la folliculo-stimuline hypophysaire (F.S.H.) diluée et dynamisée.
A.H.F. 1972.

JOUSSET P. – Expérimentation du sérum d'anguille sur le lapin.
Art médical et Bulletin de la Soc. anat., mai 1899.

JULLIAN O.A. – Psycho-pharmacologie expérimentale chez l'homme et l'animal en médecine homéopathique.
Arch. Hom. Normandie n° 35, sept. 1964.

JULLIAN O.A. – Expérimentation psycho-pathologique animale, selon les lois d'analogie et d'identité homéopathique, par la reserpine et le Cicuta-virosa.
Cahiers de Bioth. n° 9, décembre 1965.

JUNG L. – Quelques considérations physiques et physico-chimiques sur les dilutions infinitésimales.
A.H.F., 1971.

LACHARME, PICARD, BOIRON J. et FABRE. – Effets de différentes dilutions de Physotigma venenosum sur l'activité de la cholinestérase étudiée « in vitro ».
A.H.F., 1965.

LALOUETTE P. – Immunologie contemporaine et recherches homéopathiques.
A.H.F., février 1965.

LALOUETTE P. – Approche d'une démonstration expérimentale du principe de similitude.
A.H.F., juillet 1965.

LALOUETTE P. et BOYER R. – Essai de démonstration expérimentale du principe de similitude.
A.H.F., novembre 1966.

LALOUETTE P. et BOYER R. – Contribution à l'étude d'une pharmacologie homéopathique.
A.H.F., juillet 1967.

LAMASSON F. – Etude expérimentale sur l'action de dilutions Korsakoff sur des cultures de staphylocoque doré.
H.F., novembre 1945.

LAMASSON F. – Intérêt de l'étude expérimentale et projet d'étude pathogénique de certains venins non encore utilisés en homéopathie.
A.H.F., 1962.

LAMASSON F. – Réflexions à propos de la réexpérimentation d'un remède déjà étudié du temps de Hahnemann.
A.H.F., 1963.

LAMASSON F. – Notions actuellement connues sur le thallium et ses sels.
A.H.F., 1965.

LAMASSON F. – Contribution à l'étude expérimentale d'Aconitum.
A.H.F., 1965.

LAMASSON F. – Intérêt homéopathique des troubles provoqués par certains métaux récemment utilisés en métallurgie.
A.H.F., 1968.

LAPP C., WURMSER L. et KAUTRELE J. – Mobilisation du bismuth fixé chez le cobaye sous l'influence de doses infinitésimales d'un sel de bismuth.
C.H.T.C. (Cahiers d'Homéopathie et de Thérapie Comparée), 1958.

LAREBEYRETTE. – Enzymologie et conditions d'activité des doses infinitésimales.
Cah. de Bioth., décembre 1966.

LAVALL et SCHMITT. – De l'action des antibiotiques « in vitro » à dose infinitésimale.
C.H.F., 1954.

LEFEVRE N. – Etude de dilutions hahnemanniennes à l'aide de produits radioactifs.
L.M.H.I., 1976.

LUU-D., VINH. – Les dilutions homéopathiques : contrôle et étude par spectrographie Raman-Laser.
Thèse de doctorat en Pharmacie, Faculté de Montpellier, 3 juin 1974.

LUU-D. VINH, BOIRON J. – Contribution to the study of the physical structure of homeopathic dilutions by raman laser effect.
Scientific research in Homeopathy Editions Laboratoires Boiron, 1976.

LUU-D. VINH, BOIRON J. – Etude des dilutions homéopathiques par spectroscopie raman-laser.
Editions Laboratoires Boiron, 1976.

MARTINY. – Action pharmacodynamique des venins de serpent à doses infinitésimales.
Homéopathie moderne, 1938.

MASSON DE SAINT FELIX. – Données expérimentales sur le venin d'une araignée.
A.H.F., 1963.

MATHIS C. – Races chimiques chez les plantes médicinales.
A.H.F., 1971.

MOURIQUAND G., CIER A., BOIRON J., EDEL V. et CHIGHIZOLA R. – Variation de l'indice chronologique vestibulaire et de l'élimination arsenicale chez le pigeon sous l'effet de doses infinitésimales d'arsenic.
Bulletin des travaux de la Société de Pharmacie de Lyon n° 1, 1960.

MOURIQUAND G., CIER A., BOIRON J., EDEL V. et CHIGHIZOLA R. – Rétention et mobilisation de toxiques exogènes chez le pigeon.
A.H.F., 1961.

NARODETZKY. – Sur l'établissement d'une technique pour étudier les doses homéopathiques.
Thèse Université de Paris, Pharmacie, 1938.

NEBEL. – Un essai de vérification expérimentale des hautes dilutions.
Actes du Congrès Int. d'Hom. Paris 1932.

NETIEN G. – Le contrôle et l'identification des teintures-mères.
A.H.F., 1962.

NETIEN G. – Action de dilutions homéopathiques sur la respiration du coléoptile du blé.
A.H.F. n° 10, 1962.

NETIEN G. – Sur les moyens de contrôle de quelques dynamisations homéopathiques.
A.H.F., 1962.

NETIEN G. – De l'expérimentation homéopathique chez le végétal.
A.H.F., 1963.

NETIEN G. – Perspectives de recherches dans le domaine de la pharmacie homéopathique.
A.H.F., 1965.

NETIEN G. – Nouveaux tests de l'activité des doses infinitésimales.
A.H.F., 1968.

NETIEN G., BOIRON J. et MARIN A. – Action de dilutions infinitésimales de sulfate de cuivre sur des plantes préalablement intoxiquées par cette substance.
A.H.F., 1966.

NETIEN G. et GIRARDET E. – L'expérimentation des hautes dilutions dans le domaine du végétal.
A.H.F., janvier 1963.

NETIEN G., GIRARDET E. et GATTUS N. – Croissance des levures en fonction de dilutions homéopathiques hahnemanniennes.
A.H.F., 1962-1964.

NETIEN G. et GRAVIOU S. – Action d'une 5e centésimale de sulfate de cuivre sur les manifestations rythmiques de la croissance de jeunes tiges de Lepidium sativum L.
XXXIe Congrès de la L.M.H.I., Athènes, mai 1976.

PALAFER P. – Etude expérimentale de l'action des dilutions infinitésimales de « Poumon anaphylactique » sur le choc anaphylactique du cobaye.
Université Bordeaux, 1958.

PERSSON. – Travaux scientifiques d'investigation accomplis au laboratoire biochimique des médecins homéopathes de Leningrad.
Actes du Congrès int. Hom., 1932.

PERSSON. – Les doses infinitésimales en biologie et en médecine.
H.M. II, p. 469, 1933.

PERSSON. – De l'effet des microdoses homéopathiques sur la trypsine (détermination quantitative).
H.M., 1934.

PERSSON. – L'effet des microdoses médicamenteuses homéopathiques sur l'erepsine.
H.M., 1935.

PERSSON. – L'effet des microdoses de médicaments homéopathiques, substances chimiques et

d'hormones sur le ferment diastasique du muscle de grenouille.
H.M., 1936.

PICARD A. – Hypothèse sur le mode d'action des remèdes homéopathiques.
A.H.F., 1965.

PICHET. – Etude pharmacologique et physique des hautes dilutions mise au point de la question.
Actes du Congrès int. d'Hom., 1932.

PLAZY. – Intoxication professionnelle par le Béryllium.
A.H.F., 1963.

ROY. – Expérimentation de Sepia sur le cobaye femelle.
Bulletin S.F.H., 1928.

SCHNETSLER J.P. et CLEACH J. – Traitement des sensibilisations à la chlorpromazine par la chlorpromazine elle-même.
A.H.F., mai 1959.

SEVAUX F. – Contribution à l'étude biologique des hautes dilutions homéopathiques.
A.H.F., juin-juillet 1953.

SEVAUX F. – Variations des courbes électrocardiographiques après l'emploi de hautes dilutions de biothérapiques.
1er Congrès nat. méd. Hom. Rome, sept. 1957.

SEVAUX F. – Contribution à l'étude de l'action biologique des dilutions homéopathiques. Modifications de l'électrocardiogramme et remèdes homéopathiques.
Bulletin du C.H.F., 1959.

SEVAUX F. – Contribution de l'étude de l'action biologique des hautes doses homéopathiques : Psorinum 7 CH.
A.H.F., juin 1960.

SEVAUX F. – Contrôle de laboratoire de l'action biologique des dilutions homéopathiques.
A.H.F., juin 1961.

SEVAUX F. – Contribution à l'étude des hautes dilutions homéopathiques : Psorinum 7 CH.
A.H.F., janvier 1961.

SEVAUX F. – Preuves de laboratoire de l'efficacité des dilutions homéopathiques en cardiologie.
H.F., juin 1962.

SEVAUX F. – Témoins physiques de l'activité pharmacodynamique des hautes dilutions employées en homéopathie.
H.F., novembre 1963.

SEVAUX F. – Eléments de contrôle des remèdes homéopathiques par la mesure du PH, RH et résistivité électrique.
H.F., avril 1966.

SEVAUX F. – Contribution à l'étude de l'action biologique des dilutions homéopathiques.
H.F., juin 1976.

SEVAUX F. et EMAR A. – Contribution à l'étude de l'action biologique des dilutions homéopathiques : Streptococcinum 7 CH et 9 CH.
H.F., avril 1954.

SEVAUX F. et EMAR A., EMAR Mme et MAUVERNAY R.-Y. – Contribution à l'étude de l'action biologique des hautes dilutions homéopathiques.
H.F., avril 1954.

SEVAUX F., EMAR, LARCHON et ROBERT. – Contribution à l'étude de l'action biologique des hautes dilutions homéopathiques.
Bulletin du C.H.F., 1952.

SEVAUX F., EMAR, EMAR Mme et MAUVERNAY. – Contribution à l'étude de l'action biologique des hautes dilutions homéopathiques à propos d'une expérimentation de Natrum sulfuricum 7 CH.
Bulletin du C.H.F., 2e semestre, 1953.

SEVAUX F., EMAR et Collaborateurs. – Contribution à l'étude de l'action biologique des hautes dilutions homéopathiques. Trois expérimentations d'APIS 9 CH. Observations.
Bulletin du C.H.F., 2e semestre 1954.

TETAU. – Pharmacologie de Digitalis.
A.H.F., 1962.

TETAU J. et TETAU M. – Pharmacologie et psychopharmacologie de Thuya.
A.H.F., mai 1960.

TETAU et JEANNES. – Avantages et inconvénients comparés des spectres capillaires et chromatogrammes appliqués au contrôle des teintures-mères.
A.H.F., 1967.

VISCHNIAC I. – Contrôle de quelques pommades homéopathiques.
A.H.F., 1962.

VISCHNIAC I. – Influence des doses infinitésimales de plomb sur l'évolution de l'intoxication au plomb chez l'animal.
H.F., janvier 1965.

VISCHNIAC I., Mlle G. BOUNIOL. – Quelques recherches touchant le titre de l'alcool à utiliser dans la préparation des teintures-mères homéopathiques.
XIe Assises Scient. Homéo. Bordeaux, avril 1972.

WURMSER L. – Le réactif biologique dans l'étude des doses infinitésimales.
Congrès national du C.H.F., mai 1936.

WURMSER L. – La persistance de certaines actions médicamenteuses à travers les dilutions.
Congrès du C.H.F., Paris, 1938.

WURMSER L. – Action des faibles doses de Butelline sur l'intestin isolé de rat.
C.R., Soc. Biol., 1947.

WURMSER L. – Pharmacologie : un essai de pharmacologie homéopathique.
H.F., novembre-décembre 1948.

WURMSER L. – Hypothèses récentes sur le mode d'action des remèdes homéopathiques.
H.F., juillet 1949 - octobre 1949.

WURMSER L. – De l'action réciproque de différentes doses d'une même substance.
Actes des journées médicales de la Société de médecine homéopathique de l'Est (Strasbourg), 26 et 27 septembre 1953.

WURMSER L. – Action de doses infinitésimales de bismuth sur l'élimination de ce métal chez le cobaye.
H.F. n° 7, juillet 1957.

WURMSER L. – Pharmacologie et homéopathie.
Cahiers d'homéopathie et de thérapie comparée, 3e année p. 217 et congrès national de méd. Hom., Rome, 27 et 30 septembre 1957.

WURMSER L. – Réflexions pharmacologiques à propos de l'action des doses infinitésimales.
H.F., juin 1959.

WURMSER L. – Les catégories de remèdes utilisés en homéopathie.
A.H.F., 1971.

WURMSER L. – La place de l'homéopathie dans la pharmacologie contemporaine.
H.F., novembre 1973.

WURMSER L. – Preuves expérimentales de l'activité des doses infinitésimales.
Ac. Hom., 1953.

WURMSER L. – Essai de justification expérimentale de certaines aggravations médicamenteuses.
Doc. L.H.F.

WURMSER L. – Influence des doses infinitésimales sur la cinétique des éliminations.
La documentation homéopathique, n° 39.

WURMSER L. – Pathopharmacodynamie et homéopathie.
La documentation homéopathique n° 55.

WURMSER L., et LOCH P. – Recherches expérimentales sur des dilutions homéopathiques.
Congrès de la L.H.I. Budapest, 1935.

WURMSER L. et VISCHNIAC I. – Recherches sur l'action des doses infinitésimales de plomb. Essais préliminaires.
Bulletin du C.H.F., 1962.

WURMSER L. et VISCHNIAC I. – Influence de la nature du récipient sur les éléments d'identification des teintures-mères.
A.H.F., 1963.

The bibliography of more recent work will be given in a future publication.

Trials carried out in various countries

ARYA M.P. – The planning of homoeopathic research in India.
H.G., April 1976.

BODMAN Frank. – The quest for specifics.
B.H.J., 1975.

BOYD W. Hasmish. – Ideas for research in Homoeopopathy scientific and clinical.
B.H.J., October 1973.

BOYD W. Hasmish. – Biochemical and Biological Evidencies of the activity of high potencies.
B.H.J., Déc. 1954.

BRUCATO A., STEPHENSON J. – Dielectric Strength testing of Homeopathic Dilutions of $HgCl_2$.
J.A.I.H., 1966.

DANZE J.M. – Contribution à l'étude analytique de certaines substances d'origine animale.
R.B.H., n° 1, 1974.

DELESTINNE. – Recherches anciennes en homéopathie.
R.B.H. n° 3, 1975.

DEMERBE Marie-Yvonne. – Observations sur l'action de quelques venins de serpents et de crapaud sur les souris blanches, corrélations avec les pathogénésies existantes.
R.B.H. n° 4, 1975.

DESAI. – Some experiences with strychnine, Ars. and Plumbum met.
B.H.J., July 1969.

DOUCH G. – Granulocyte reactions after homeopathic potencies.
B.H.J., April 1966.

DUTTA A.C. – Experiments with inorganic nutrients in Homoeopathic dilution on plants and existence of micro isotopes.
H.G., Oct. 1976.

GIBSON M. – Nitricum acidum, a study.
B.H.J., April 1972.

JENAER M. – Essai de prévention d'un cancer expérimental par les acides nucléiques dynamisés.
R.B.H., March 1976.

JENAER M. – Essai de prévention de la leucémie lymphoide spontanée de la souris AKR par ARN-ADN dynamisés.
R.B.H., 1977.

KAHN M.T. – Estimation of low and high potencies of Aconit by means of biochemical methods.

KAHN M.T. – Topics and methods for homeopathic research.
Cong. L.M.H.I., 1975.

KAHN M.T., Z.S. SAIFY. – Physical aspects related to the problems in potentized drugs.
Cong. L.M.H.I., 1973.

KAHN M.T., Z.S. SAIFY. – Physical aspects to the problem in low and high homeopathic potentized drugs.
Cong. L.M.H.I., 1973.

KOFFLER WANNAMAKER. – Effects of Boron Dynamizations on Onions.
J.A.I.H., 1967.

NOIRET R. et GLAUDE M. – Etude enzymatique du grain de froment intoxique par CuSO4 et traité par différentes dilutions hahnemanniennes de la même substance.
R.B.H., 1976.

NOIRET R. et Glaude M. – Activité de diverses dilutions homéopathiques de CuSO4 sur quelques souches microbiennes.
Cong. L.M.H.I., 1976.

RAWSON. – A scientific approach to Homoeopathy.
B.H.J., 1972.

RAWSON. – On the nature of serial dilution and succussion with a note on homoeopathic provings.
H.G., Dec. 1976.

SEITSCHEK. – Des rapports entre les hautes dilutions homéopathiques et les réactions granulocytiques.
Arch. Hom. Normandie, avril 1963.

SCHWARSHAUPT. – Notions de macro et microtoxicologie découlant des essais de médicaments homéopathiques.
Congrès d'Amsterdam, septembre 1961.

SMITH jr. – Research report June 1969-July 1970.
J.A.I.H., 1971.

SMITH R.B., BOERICKE G.W. – Modern Instrumentation for the evaluation of Homeopathic drug structure.
J.A.I.H., 1966.

SMITH R.B., BOERICKE G.W. – Changes caused by succussion on NMR Patterns and Biossay of bradykinintriacetat (BTK) succussions and dilutions.
J.A.I.H., 1968.

SMITH R.B. jr, BOERICKE G.W. – Continued research with modern instrumentation for the evaluation of homeopathic drug structure.
J.A.I.H., 1976.

STEPHENSON J. – A review of investigations into the action of substances in dilutions greater then L.E-24.
J.A.I.H., 1955.

VINCENT VANDEN ABEELE Sylviane. – Quelques preuves expérimentales de l'activité des remèdes homéopathiques.
R.B.H., June and Sept. 1975.

Articles taken from "Allgemeine Homöopathische Zeitung"
(from 1948 to 1976)

1948, N° 193
Toxikologische Beiträge zur homöopathischen Arzneimittelprüfung - A. Göricke.
Beitrag zur Methodik der hom. Arzneimittelprüfung - H. Schoeler.
Toxikologische Beiträge zur hom. Arzneimittelprüfung - O. Gener.

1949, N° 194
Toxikologische Beiträge zur hom. Arzneimittelprüfung - Dr. Croneberg.
Konstitution und Arzneiprüfung - A. Stiegele.

1950, N° 195
Das Hochpotenzproblem - H. Schoeler.
Toxikologische Beiträge zur hom. Arzneimittelprüfung - H. Strigel.
Homöopathie in neueren Arzneimitteln und neuere Arzneimittel in der Homöopathie - H. Schoeler.

1951, N° 196
Über gewerbliche Zinkschädigung und ihre Beziehung zur hom. Arzneimittellehre - H. Ritter.
Beitrag zur Chemie, Pharmakologie und Klinik der Mistel (Viscum album) - H. Skroka.
Toxikologische Beiträge zur hom. Arzneimittelprüfung (Spinnenbisse, Strychnin etc).
Beitrag zur Arzneiwirkung der Asa foetida - A. Stiegele.
Toxikologie und Homöopathie - H. Ortloff.
Neuere Arzneiprüfungen von Bryonia - E. Unseld.

1952, N° 197
Chlornatrium und die Reizpathophysiologie - H. von Ritter (Übersetzer Jacques Duflo)
Toxikologische Beiträge - Über die Giftwirkung des Tannin.
Die Beziehungen der Akupunktur, der Weihelschen Druckpunkte und der Neuraltherapie zur Homöopathie - H. Schoeler.

1953, N° 198
Synergie in der Homöopathie-dargestellt an Beispielen aus der Veterinärmedizin - H. Wolter.

1954, N° 199
Die Bedeutung neuer Funktionspathologischer Erkenntnisse für die Homöopathie - H. Schoeler.
Toxikologische Beiträge zur hom. Arzneimittellehere - H. Ortloff - Penicillin-homöopathische gesehen.
Über physikalische Wirkungen oder Eigenschaften echter hom. Hochpotenzen - H. Schoeler.
Die Reproduzierbarkeit der Simileregel in der Therapie am Beispiel der Bryonia - P. Mössinger.
Erkrankungen durch Mangan und seine Verbindungen - K. Sroka.
Aristolochia innerhalb der Sterilitätsbehandlung der Grosstiere - H. Wolter.

1955, N° 200
Toxikologische Beiträge- Ammoniakvergiftungen der oberen Luftwege - A. Kühne.
Neuere Ergebnisse der franz. Hom. auf dem Gebiet des Hochpotenzproblems.
Erfahrungen mit Arnica montana und Belladonna parenteral bei mehreren Hochdruckfällen und apoplektischen Insulten.
Neuartige Darstellung hom. Arzneimittelbilder - R. Schur-Rieve.
Taraxacum officinale - W. Pischel.
AMP von Carcinosin (zusammengefasster Bericht).

1956, N° 201
Der derzeitige Stand der Arbeiten zum Nachweis der Hochpotenzen - Aper. E. Scholz.
Beiträge zur Pharmakodynamik nach homöopathischen Prinzipien - Dr. Lobethal.
Zur Hochpotenzfrage - H. Schoeler.
Zum Hochpotenzproblem - J. Zinke.
Belladonna (Zusammenfassung Angabe von AMP) - O. Leeser.

1957, N° 202
Bericht über eine Versuchsreihe mit Berberis aquifolium (Mahonie) - H. Unger.

1958, N° 203
Die Homöopathie im Licht der modernen Naturwissenschaft - E. Unseld.
Zum Arzneimittelbild des Besenginsters - M. Stübler.
Cantharis - Bericht über eine unbeabsichtigte Arzneiprüfung - J. Zinke.

Betrachtungen über die Besenginsterzubereitungen unter besonderer Berücksichtigung der homöopath. Urtinktur - H. Schindler.

Der Gebungsbereich des Arndt-Schulzschen Saltzes - G. Bayr.

Das Simileprinzip in moderner Sicht - W. Zimmermann.

Ein Beitrag zur Kenntnis von Vergiftung mit Barium - Z. Maretic, J. Homadowvski, S. Razbojnkov, V. Brecevic.

Iberis amara (eine Arzneimittelprüfung) - R. Jehn.

Cadmium metallicum - W. Gutmann.

Asa foetida - H. Unger.

Arzneimittelprüfung mit Cobaltum nitricum - G. Marin.

Beryllium - W. Gutmann.

Über den wissenschaftlichen Wert der hom. Arzneiprüfungen - A.J. Gruber.

Das Arzneibild Peyotl - H. Unger.

1959, N° 204

Homöopathie und Tierversuche - H. Wolter.

1960 - N° 205

Eine Arzneimittelprüfung mit dem Besenginster-Sarothamnus scoparius - J. Mezger - M. Stübler.

1961, N° 206

Eine Prüfung von Hydrophis cyanocinctus - J.R. Raeside.

Arzneimittelprüfung un Allergie - A. Hollenberg.

Eine Arzneimittelprüfung mit Dichapetalum - G. Maring.

Die Methodik der Arzneimittelprüfung in der Homöopathie - J. Mezger.

Vergleichende Betrachtung der Arzneimittelbilder der Spinnen - J. Mezger.

Arzneimittelprüfung und Allergie - A. Hollenberg.

1962, N° 207

Über die Nachprüfung von Belladonna - R. Stengel.

Eine Arzneimittelprüfung mit Bryonia - R. Pirtkien - Hippokrates - Verlag (Veröffentlichungen aus dem RBK).

Die hom. Arzneimittelprüfung vom pathophysiologischen Standpunkt aus - E. Unseld.

Beryllium - Symptomenbild - H. Wirsam.

Zur Pharmakodynamik und Pharmakotherapie des Nitroglycerins - E. Unseld.

Zur Pharmakologie des Placebo - H. Haas.

Viperatoxin und Kobratoxin, Toxikologie und homöotherapeutische Folgerungen G.R. Kerl.

Altes und Neues über Jod und Fluor - J. Mezger.

Die Möglichkeiten makro- und mikrotoxikologischer Erkenntnisse in ihrem Verhältnis zur hom. Arzneimittelprüfung - W. Schwarzhaupt.

Angewandte Arzneimittelprüfung bei Tieren in neuralpathologischen Zusammenhang - H. Wolter.

Speicherung und Mobilisierung exogener Gifte bei der Taube - G. Mouriquand.

Die homöop. Arzneimittelprüfung im Spiegel-causalanalytische und anthropologischer Betrachtungsweise - F. Donner.

1963, N° 208

Nachweisbare hom. Arzneiwirkungen akuter Krankheitszustände bei Tieren, insbes. Schweinen - H. Wolter.

Studie zum Capsicumbild - W. Zimmermann.

Toxikologie, Pharmakologie und Therapie der Solanumgruppe - W. Zimmermann.

Bryonia im doppelten Blindversuch - J. Mezger.

Eine Arzneimittelprüfung mit Belladonna - R. Pirtkien - Hippokrates Verlag (Veröffentlichungen aus dem RBK).

1964, N° 209

Flor de Piedra - W. Schwabe und W. Herz.

Therapieerfahrungen mit Flor de Piedra - E. Freiwald.

Die Realität der Arzneimittelbilder - R. Richwien.

Mandragora - Arzneibild und Erfahrungen - J. Mezger.

Belladonna-Wirkung bei Haustieren - H. Wolter.

1965, N° 210

Experimentelle Untersuchungen über die Kreislaufwirkung von Veratrum album - H. Schoeler.

1966, N° 211

Arzneiwirkungsprüfung an Caulophyllum D30 - H. Wolter.

Gesichtspunkte zur Darstellung der hom. Arzneimittelbilder - J. Mezger.

Biophysik der homoepathischen Arzneiwirkung - F. Kracmar.

1967, N° 212

Gedanken zu einer neuen Darstellungsform von Arzneimittelbildern - H. Unger.

Klinischer Kurzbeitrag zur Wirksamkeit von Lespedeza Sieboldi - J. Wunderli.

Galphimia glaucaein neues antispezifisches Antiallergicum - W. Herz.

Über eine unfreiwillige Arzneimittelprüfung mit Arsen - K.H. Illing.

1968, N° 213

Zur Frage der Arzneimittelprüfung in unserer Zeit - H. Schoeler.

Zur Frage der Wirksamkeit potenzierter Substanzen - E. Friedrich.

Experimentelle Untersuchungen über die Leberwirksamkeit von Flor de Piedra - H. Wolter.

Luffa operculata, ein nach homöop. Gesichtspunkten neu aufgefundenes Mittel bei Krankheiten im Nasen-Rachenraum.

1969,

Weitere Erfahrungen mit Flor de Piedra - H. Wolter.

Toxikologische Beiträge zur Arzneimittelprüfung - W. Pischel.

1970, N° 215

Molekulargenetik und hom. Konstitutionstherapie - H. Beuchelt.

Eine neue Arzneimittelprüfung mit Asarum europaeum - J. Mezger.

Toxikologische Beiträge zur homöopathischen Arzneimittelprüfung - W. Pischel.

1971, N° 216

Über eine neue Arzneimittelprüfung von Cimicifuga racemosa - J. Mezger.

Behandlung des Schleimbeutelhygroms mit Apis - P. Nössinger.

Die Anwendung der Harpagophytum-Wurzel bei rheumatischen Erkrankungen - A. Beham.

1972, N° 217

Eine Arzneimittelprüfung von Espeletia grandiflora - W. Klunker.

Espeletia grandiflora - M. Stübler - Kasuistik.

Anacardium orientale - E.H. Schmeer.

Okoubaka, ein neues homöopathisches Arzneimittel - M. Kunst.

Erste Erfahrungen mit einigen exotischen Heilpflanzen in homöopathischer Verarbeitung - W. Schwabe.

1973, N° 218

Über die Wasserhyazinthe-Eichhornia crassipies - H. Schoeler.

Toxikologische Beiträge zur homöop. Arzneimittelprüfung - W. Pischel.

Behandlung des Schleimbeutelhygroms mit Apis - P. Mössinger.

Die Behandlung der Pharyngitis mit Phytolacca - P. Mössinger.

Die Behandlung des Ganglions mit Silicea - P. Mössinger.

Myrtillocactus geometrizans - G. Kampik.

Einführung in das homöop. Arzneipotenzierungsverfahren - E. Unseld.

1974, N° 219

Gedanken zur systematischen Erfassung den Wirkungen homöop. Arzneimittel am Menschen - K. Kleinschmidt.

Eine Neuprüfung mit Magnesium muriaticum - J. Mezger.

Über meine Erfahrungen mit Arzneimittelprüfungen - J. Mezger.

Sanguinaria beim Kopfschmerz - H. Ritter.

Prüfungssymptome in der Praxis - K.H. Illing.

1975, N° 220

Über Lachesis - H. Ritter.

1976, N° 221

Eine Arzneimittelprüfung mit Adlumia fungosa - G. Bayr.

Eine Arzneimittelprüfung mit Asterias rubens - J. Mezger.

Erfahrungen mit FdP D3 in der tierärztlichen Praxis - W. Greiff.

ACHEVÉ D'IMPRIMER
SUR LES PRESSES
DE COMIMPRIM
69002 LYON FRANCE

LABORATOIRES BOIRON
20, RUE DE LA LIBÉRATION
69110 SAINTE-FOY-LÈS-LYON

ISBN 2.85742.011.0 - Dépôt légal n° 993 - Janvier 1984